Workbook to Accompany *Fundamentals of Basic Emergency Care*

Second Edition

Richard W. O. Beebe, MEd, RN, NREMT-P
Program Director
Bassett Healthcare
Center for Rural Emergency Medical Services Education
Cooperstown, New York

Adjunct Faculty
Herkimer County Community College
Herkimer, New York

Deborah L. Funk, MD, NREMT-P
Instructor
Emergency Medicine
Albany Medical College
Albany, New York

Attending Physician
Emergency Department
Albany Medical Center Hospital
Albany, New York

Written by
Deborah Kufs, MS, RN, NREMT-P
Clinical Coordinator
Institute for Prehospital Emergency Medicine
Hudson Valley Community College
Troy, New York

THOMSON
DELMAR LEARNING™

Australia Canada Mexico Singapore Spain United Kingdom United States

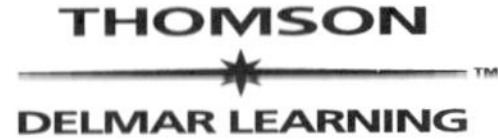

Workbook to Accompany

***Fundamentals of Basic Emergency Care,* Second Edition**

by Richard W. O. Beebe and Deborah L. Funk

Written by Deborah Kufs

Vice President, Health Care Business Unit:
William Brottmiller

Editorial Director:
Cathy L. Esperti

Acquisitions Editor:
Maureen Rosener

Senior Developmental Editor:
Darcy M. Scelsi

Editorial Assistant:
Elizabeth Howe

Marketing Director:
Jennifer McAvey

Marketing Coordinator:
Christopher Manion

Art and Design Specialist:
Jack Pendleton

Production Coordinator:
Anne Sherman

Project Editor:
David Buddle

Printed in the United States of America
1 2 3 4 5 6 7 XXX 08 07 06 05 04

For more information, contact Thomson Delmar Learning, 5 Maxwell Drive, Clifton Park, NY 12065
Or find us on the World Wide Web at http://www.delmarlearning.com.

ISBN 1-4018-7934-9

NOTICE TO THE READER

Dedication

For Bob, whose belief in me is never-ending.
To Genna and Kim, firefighters and paramedics.
To Matt, the light of my life.
—DLK

Contents

Preface

This workbook was designed to accompany *Fundamentals of Basic Emergency Care,* Second Edition. Exercises designed to help you review text material, key terms, and skills are provided. This workbook was designed to allow a step-by-step progression of learning: from understanding terminology to learning discrete skills and concepts to applying the material.

Prehospital emergency care is a combination of thinking and doing. The workbook material challenges you to acquire the basic knowledge, use critical thinking skills, and develop the hands-on skills necessary for practice as an EMT–Basic.

Regulations covering the practice of prehospital emergency care vary from state to state; therefore, it is important for you to learn the specific regulation in your area.

Further supplement your review of the content in the text and workbook by using the StudyWare™ CD-ROM provided in your text. The StudyWare software helps you learn concepts discussed in *Fundamentals of Basic Emergency Care,* Second Edition. As you study each chapter in the text, be sure to explore the activities in the corresponding chapter in the software. CD icons in the text indicate that there is related content on the CD-ROM. Use StudyWare as your own private tutor to help you learn the material in your text. Included in StudyWare are:

- Quizzes with multiple choice, true or false, fill-in, and word building questions
- Activities such as image labeling and a "Jeopardy" style championship game
- Multimedia consisting of animations and video clips related to content you have studied in the text
- Web links to research topics on your own and give you resources for additional information on topics covered in each chapter
- Possible solutions to the cases in the text to help you fine-tune your critical thinking and problem-solving skills

CHAPTER 1 Introduction to Emergency Medical Services

EMTs are the foundation of the prehospital component of emergency medical services. This review will assist you in recalling historical events and reflecting upon their implications for your new vocation.

Matching: Match each word or term with its definition.

1. ____ first responders
2. ____ EMT–Basic
3. ____ EMT–Intermediate
4. ____ EMT–Paramedic
5. ____ EMD
6. ____ IAFF
7. ____ NHTSA
8. ____ Star of Life
9. ____ emergency physician
10. ____ white paper

a. national EMS symbol
b. laid the groundwork for inclusion of EMS in federal legislation
c. a national level of care that involves administering oxygen and simple bleeding control
d. a doctor trained to give care to the acutely ill or injured
e. represents the fire service
f. a method of questioning callers and giving lifesaving instructions
g. most common prehospital provider
h. a branch of the Department of Transportation
i. highest level of prehospital provider
j. provider trained in advanced airway management and IV therapy

True or False: Read each statement and decide if it is true or false. Place T or F on the line before each statement.

1. _____ Providing care to the sick or injured can be traced back to ancient times.
2. _____ Modern emergency medical service is designed only for lifesaving care.
3. _____ The military had little involvement in the development of modern EMS.
4. _____ The American Red Cross was formed by Deke Farrington.
5. _____ The "white paper" was written to describe death in the Vietnam War.
6. _____ OSHA was formed to meet the needs of EMTs, and to speak to the public about EMS.
7. _____ Universal Access is designed so that all emergency services can be reached by a three-digit number.
8. _____ Emergency medical dispatch consists of lifesaving phone instructions and triage.
9. _____ EMT-Bs work only on ambulances.
10. _____ Paramedics are the highest trained prehospital care providers.

Short Answer: Read each question. Think about the information presented in your text, and then answer each question with one or two sentences.

1. The concept of the *ambulances volante* is still practiced today. From the text, give an example.

2. Why did soldiers in Vietnam have a greater chance for survival than drivers and pedestrians in the United States?

3. Johnny and Roy led the American public to think differently about people suffering illnesses or injuries before they could get to a hospital. What did this change in thinking do for health care?

4. What components are necessary for a successful "EMS chain of survival"?

5. Which of these components is influenced by the EMT-B?

6. How is EMS provided in your community?

7. What changes do you expect to see in the future of EMS?

8. How do the various prehospital care providers, communicators, physicians, and allied health professionals contribute to the concepts drawn from the Star of Life?

CHAPTER 2
Medical Responsibilities

The EMT-B provides medical care to patients in many different settings. Responsibility for safety, quality care, and adhering to standards belongs to the EMT-B when providing medical care.

Ordering: Place the following duties in the order in which they should be performed for a call. Put a numeral 1 before the first duty, a 2 before the next, and so on.

_____ Assess patient

_____ Call medical control as needed

_____ Continue care during transport

_____ Determine mechanism of injury or nature of illness

_____ Drive safely to scene

_____ Give verbal and written reports to staff

_____ Replace any equipment used

_____ Move patient to the ambulance

_____ Notify destination facility of patient

_____ Perform scene assessment

_____ Reassess patient

_____ Receive information from dispatch

Identification: Place an X in front of those patient-care responsibilities performed by EMT-Bs.

_____ Airway maintenance

_____ Ventilation of patients

_____ Intubation of patients

_____ CPR

_____ Defibrillation by AED

_____ Manual cardioversion

_____ Hemorrhage control

_____ Suturing of wounds

_____ Bandaging of wounds

_____ Assisting in childbirth

_____ Prescribing medications to patients

True or False: Read each statement and decide if it is true or false. Place T or F on the line before each statement.

1. _____ The first priority of any EMT-B is personal safety.
2. _____ Good safety precautions always involve complicated procedures.
3. _____ EMT-Bs should never remove a patient from a dangerous situation until medical care has been provided.
4. _____ Continuing medical education is necessary for EMT-Bs.
5. _____ After the EMT-B takes a state written exam, she will be licensed to practice in that state.
6. _____ Quality management is an administrative role performed by the agency's top administrative officer.
7. _____ Retrospective quality assessment is performed by a team member accompanying the crews on calls.

Definitions: Write the definitions of the following terms.

1. certification ______________________________
2. medical direction ______________________________
3. off-line medical control ______________________________
4. on-line medical control ______________________________
5. quality management ______________________________
6. professional conduct ______________________________
7. quality improvement ______________________________
8. prehospital health care team ______________________________

Identification: Read each of the following statements and determine if it describes classroom (didactic), hands-on (psychomotor), or clinical (integration) opportunity. Place the correct word on the line in front of the statement.

1. ______________ The instructor assigns readings from the text.
2. ______________ The student completes medical rounds with an emergency physician.
3. ______________ A student is moulaged (made up), while another assesses for injuries.
4. ______________ A case study is presented, and the class describes care.
5. ______________ A student observes and plans care while riding with an EMT-B on an ambulance.

Short Answer: Read each question. Think about the information presented in your text, and then answer each question with one or two sentences.

1. Why is it important for the EMT to reassure bystanders during a call?

2. Explain the value of a clean identifiable uniform and name tag.

3. Why must the EMT-B consider added training after her initial course?

Critical Thinking 1: Read the following case study and then answer the questions.

Jenna, Kimberley, and Andy were called to the home of an older female patient who had difficulty breathing. After the call was completed and the ambulance restocked, they stopped for a well-deserved meal at the local diner. The EMTs were annoyed that a woman would continue to smoke, even after her doctor had advised her not to do so. They talked amongst themselves about the patient, her obvious lack of commitment to taking care of herself, and their resentment at being called frequently just "because she won't listen to her doctor."

1. Based on the EMT Code of Ethics, what did the EMTs in this study violate?

2. How would you feel if the patient in this scenario were your relative?

3. Based on the Code of Ethics, what actions could the EMTs take in promoting a healthier lifestyle choice?

Critical Thinking 2: Read the following case study and then answer the questions.

The captain of the ambulance squad was frustrated. Four times in the last month, patients were dropped off at the hospital without immobilization of swollen, deformed, painful extremities. Nothing in the run reports indicated that a more pressing need was assigned priority, and to make things worse, nothing even indicated that the injuries were found and assessed! Something had to change!

1. What five elements must be performed to ensure the ultimate goal of quality medical care?

2. What two forms of assessment are available to team members in evaluating the care that was given?

3. Which of these has the captain of the ambulance squad used?

4. Based on quality management elements, suggest a way in which the captain can help promote improvements in care for patients with injured extremities.

Critical Thinking 3: Read the following case study and then answer the questions.

Bonnie and Howard answered a call for a man who had been stung by a bee. When they arrived, he told them that he had been stung several times while in his backyard and was now having some trouble breathing. He said that he had a history of allergy to stings and had an EpiPen prescribed, but that it was in his coat pocket and he couldn't get to it. Howard obtained the EpiPen as Bonnie completed an initial assessment and got a set of vital signs. Based on the procedures in their community, they assisted the man in self-injecting the medication. They continued with oxygen administration and transported the man to the hospital for evaluation. During transport, they reassessed him, and Howard spoke with the physician at the receiving hospital. He received orders to administer oxygen by a different device. The patient was dropped off at the hospital. A week after this call, the agency's medical director reviewed the call with Howard and Bonnie, complimenting them on a job well done, and making a suggestion for improvement in the future.

1. Which actions are based on off-line medical control?

2. Which are based on on-line medical control?

3. In what way did Howard and Bonnie act as the physician's designated agent?

CHAPTER 3 The Legal Responsibilities of the EMT

Emergency medical service is considered a public trust. The public expects prompt, professional care plus attention to individual rights.

Completion: Complete the missing word or words in each sentence.

1. A__ __ __ __ __ __ __ __ __ __t is leaving a patient who is in your care unsupervised.
2. A breach of __ __ __ f i __ __ __ __ __ __ __ __ __ __ __ occurs when a person divulges information about another without permission.
3. An awareness of the importance of preserving evidence at the scene of a crime constitutes e__ __ __e__ __ __ c o__ __ __ __ __ __ __ __.
4. __ __ __ __ S__ __ __ __ __ __ __ __n __ __ __s were designed to protect certain classes of people when they are helping others.
5. H__ __ __ __ __ c__ __ __ p__ __ __ __ enables a person to make care decisions for someone who is not capable of doing so.
6. A presumption that a person would agree to be treated if she could agree defines i__ __ __ __ __ __ c__ __ __ __ __ __.
7. A person required by law to take a particular action has a l__ __ __ __ d__ __ __ to a__ __.
8. Written instructions for an EMT is part of __ __ __ __ __ __ __ __ medical control.
9. Speaking with the doctor on the radio is part of __ __ __ __ __ __ medical control.
10. The patient's __ __ __ __ of __ __ __ __ __ __ are what the patient expects when being cared for in a hospital or health facility.
11. A group of injuries common to a certain mechanism is called a p__ __ __ __ __ __ __ of __ __ __ __ __ __ __.
12. Restriction of a patient's freedom by ties or cravats is called physical __ __ __ __ __ __ __ __ __.
13. An action or inaction that is the direct reason for harm is termed c__ __ __ __ __ __ __ __ __ of i__ __ __ __ __.
14. The level of care recognized as being required is a __ __ __ __ __ __ __ __ of care.
15. __ __ __ __ __ regulations require protected health information to be held in strict confidence.

Identification: Read the following and determine the type of consent in each case. Write the type on the line in front of the case.

1. ____________ When the EMT tells Mrs. Jones that he needs to obtain a blood pressure reading, she rolls up her sleeve and holds out her arm.
2. ____________ The school nurse gives permission for the EMT to examine a child injured on the playground.
3. ____________ The EMTs assess a man who is unconscious. He is at the mall and no one is with him.
4. ____________ The police ask the EMT to assess a severely injured man they are arresting.
5. ____________ The EMTs provide care to a child who is choking and cannot breathe.
6. ____________ Mr. Jones tells the EMTs that he called 9-1-1 because he couldn't breathe well.

7. ____________ Mrs. Brown gives permission for the EMT to bandage a cut on her 3-year-old daughter's arm.
8. ____________ While home from the army, 17-year-old Jeff gives permission for the EMT to assess him after a motor vehicle collision.

True or False: Read each statement and decide if it is true or false. Place T or F on the line before each statement.

1. _____ Apnea (not breathing) is considered a sign of irreversible death.
2. _____ Lividity can be reversed with adequate oxygenation.
3. _____ Decapitation is defined as severing of the head from the body.
4. _____ A mortal wound means the patient can survive her injuries with routine care.
5. _____ A DNR means that the EMT cannot treat the patient without a direct physician's order.
6. _____ A living will expresses the patient's wishes in regard to prolonging life.
7. _____ EMTs are not involved in the care of patients dying from a terminal illness.
8. _____ Stiffening of the muscles after death is called decomposition.

Identification: Circle the five elements in a malpractice case that must be proved for the EMT to be liable for negligence.

standard of care	a criminal action
protocols	allegations
duty to act	harm
a mistake	causation of injury
a failure to meet standards	

Yes or No: Read each of the following statements and decide if the EMTs can disclose the patient information or not. Write YES if they can, or NO if they cannot do so legally.

1. _____ A police officer asks if the patient admitted to smoking marijuana.
2. _____ A doctor who is a friend of the patient's father asks what the patient's chief complaint is.
3. _____ An emergency department nurse asks for the patient's vital signs.
4. _____ Witnesses to an accident ask if the patient is the school superintendent.
5. _____ An insurance adjuster asks the EMTs if the accident was caused by the patient.
6. _____ A surgeon called by the emergency physician asks about the patient's position in the vehicle.
7. _____ The patient's mother asks if her daughter admitted to being pregnant.
8. _____ A lawyer asks to read the patient care report.
9. _____ A nurse at the hospital asks if you transported her friend to the emergency department.
10. _____ The physician's assistant asks for a list of the patient's medications for the emergency department chart.

Identification: Place an X in front of the appropriate behaviors when dealing with a crime scene.

_____ Keep unnecessary people off the scene

_____ Use the patient's telephone to avoid radio communications

_____ Leave all medical materials on the scene

Turn off lights

_____ Remember anything that must be moved for patient care

_____ Do not touch weapons

_____ Leave answering machines or caller identification devices alone

_____ Cover the body to maintain modesty

_____ Do not use the sink to wash hands

_____ Turn off the TV, radio, and video equipment

Short Answer: Read each question. Think about the information presented in your text, and then answer each question with one or two sentences.

1. What conditions must be identified before a patient can be allowed to refuse medical assistance?

2. Explain the value of good listening skills when a patient is refusing medical care or assistance.

Critical Thinking 1: Read the following case study and then answer the questions.

Sixteen-year-old Amy and her boyfriend, Aaron, have had sexual relations on several occasions. Amy has been feeling sick lately and is concerned that she may be pregnant or have developed symptoms of a disease. At her clinic visit, Amy signs her own consent form.

1. Why can the clinic accept Amy's consent for assessment and treatment?

2. List other circumstances in which an EMT could accept consent from a minor.

Critical Thinking 2: Read the following case study and then answer the questions.

Brenda and Jeff have been dispatched to a home for a 60-year-old man who is having chest pressure. The man, Mr. Rotelli, appears ill as they enter the residence. His wife has called EMS even though the patient is saying that this is the result of too much sausage and peppers the night before. Mr. Rotelli tells the EMTs that he doesn't need to go to the hospital.

1. What should the EMTs say to Mr. Rotelli?

2. If Mr. Rotelli still doesn't want to go to the hospital, what should they do next?

3. What must be documented regarding Mr. Rotelli's refusal?

Critical Thinking 3: Read the following case study and then answer the question.

Andrew and Dory are called to the home of a 65-year-old female patient who has a history of breast cancer. Mr. Johnson called EMS because his wife was in pain. When the EMTs arrive, they find Mrs. Johnson slumped over on the couch. Initial assessment shows her not to be breathing and without a pulse. As Dory prepares to begin CPR, Andrew says he will grab the defibrillator. Mr. Johnson tells them to please stop as his wife doesn't want anything like that. She has a DNR order, but he doesn't know where it is.

1. What should Dory and Andrew do next?

Critical Thinking 4: Read the following case study and then answer the questions.

Kandy and Tom arrive on the scene of a 5-year-old boy who has a leg injury. The little boy won't talk to them or to his parents, who tell the EMTs that their son fell off the swing set several hours ago. The little boy, Jason, ignores the EMTs as they attempt to assess his leg and find out where it hurts. His parents then tell the EMTs that Jason knew he shouldn't have been on the slide and that they knew he would hurt himself someday.

1. What should the EMTs observe about the parents and child?

2. What should Kandy and Tom report to the emergency department staff?

CHAPTER 4 Stress in Emergency Medical Services

The EMT-B will be faced with many emotional and stressful situations. These situations can cause physical and emotional reactions. The EMT-B must recognize the common stressors and plan to handle them effectively.

Missing Letters: Complete the puzzle using the Key Terms in Chapter 4 of the textbook.

_ _ _ _ **s** _ _ _ _ _ _ _ _ _ isolation

_ _ _ **t** _ stress

_ _ **r** _ out

stress _ _ _ _ _ _ _ **e** _ _ program

healthy _ _ _ _ **s** _ _ _ _

scene **s** _ _ _ _ _

st**r** _ _ _ _ _ _

relaxation **e** _ _ _ _ _ _ _ _ _

multiple _ _ **s** _ _ _ _ _ incident

fight or _ _ _ _ _ _ _ _ _ _ **p** _ _ _ _

_ _ _ **o** _ _ _ stress

_ **n** _ _ _ _ time

_ _ _ _ _ **s**

diversionary _ _ _ _ _ _ _ _ **e** _

Matching: Match each word or term with its definition.

1. ____ stress
2. ____ stressors
3. ____ fight or flight response
4. ____ unwind time
5. ____ healthy lifestyle
6. ____ burnout
7. ____ acute stress
8. ____ chronic stress

a. a single event that causes a stress reaction
b. physical, emotional, behavioral response of the body to changing conditions
c. exercise, balanced diet, no smoking
d. events that trigger stress
e. opportunity to relax
f. repeated events affecting the EMT over time
g. condition that arises from chronic stress
h. response of the body to stress by preparing to run or defend itself

Sorting: Read each of the following and determine if it describes physical, emotional, or behavioral signs of chronic stress exposure. Place the word or phrase under the correct category.

alcohol abuse	gastrointestinal distress
aggression	headaches
anger	increased heart rate
anxiety	insomnia
avoidance	irritability
depression	muscle tension
drug abuse	procrastination
edgy	withdrawal
fatigue	

Physical	**Emotional**	**Behavioral**

Short Answer: Read each question. Think about the information presented in your text, and then answer each question with one or two sentences.

1. Why would prevention of stressful situations be preferable to treating stress reactions?

2. List two ways in which EMTs can decrease the number of encounters with high stress situations.

Critical Thinking 1: Read each of the following and think of a way that the perception can be changed. Write your answer below.

1. Jaime is angry because the nurse in the ED didn't answer her question.

2. Ginny is scared to begin her new job as an EMT-B.

3. Patrick can't sleep after a call in which a man with cancer died in the ambulance.

4. Greg develops a queasy feeling whenever he brings a patient to the cardiac cath lab.

Critical Thinking 2: Read the following case study and then answer the questions.

Liz had been practicing as an EMT for several years when she decided to return to school and become a paramedic. It was hard work, but her colleagues supported her efforts. Today was the big day; she expected her test results in the mail. As expected, she scored well and would be on her way to different responsibilities. Her coworkers were cheering when Liz broke down in tears and said she had no interest in being a paramedic.

1. Could Liz be experiencing stress? Why or why not?

2. How could Liz alter the perception of this event?

Critical Thinking 3: Read the following case study and then answer the questions.

Geoff had finally finished a long shift. There were many calls in the previous 24 hours, and most had involved both physical care of the patient and much explanation to each family. One gentleman had suffered from chest pain, and his family had difficulty understanding the need for an oxygen mask. A young child had been found lethargic and ill this morning, and the doctors think she may have meningitis. Geoff may even need some medications to prevent him from developing the illness. Two youngsters were playing by the road and one suffered an arm injury after being hit by a car. The shift went on and on. When Geoff arrived home, he discovered that his wife had given their 4-year-old son some medication for a fever. Geoff became very angry and upset. He started yelling at his wife and even screamed at the dog.

1. From the case study, list at least five events that may be stressful for Geoff.

2. List five diversionary techniques that may help Geoff manage stress.

Critical Thinking 4: Read the following case study and then answer the questions.

Mr. Linkowski was being transported to the dialysis facility for the third treatment this week. He was very quiet but did mention that he wouldn't be seeing the crew next week as he knew that he would not live through the weekend. Janice, the EMT, tried to cheer him up but only succeeded in making herself feel worse. Back at the station, she complained of feeling sick to her stomach and having a headache.

1. What is the likely cause of Janice's illness?

2. Suggest a reason for this to occur.

3. How can Janice change her perception of this event?

Critical Thinking 5: Read the following case study and then answer the questions.

The Midtown Ambulance Service was dispatched to a motor vehicle collision in front of the high school. The media were already there. The collision was relatively minor, didn't involve any of the school kids, and could be handled by only one ambulance crew. Joe, an EMT who had participated in a much more severe call in front of the high school in his hometown, kept yelling that they should get more ambulances ready and get the cameras out of his way.

1. What is the likely cause of Joe's reaction?

2. What are some of the signs that Joe's crew members should be aware of regarding Joe's behavior?

CHAPTER 5
Anatomy and Physiology

To understand a patient's illness or injury, the EMT-B must have a basic understanding of human anatomy and physiology.

Matching: Match each word or term with its definition.

1. ____ anatomy
2. ____ physiology
3. ____ standard anatomic position
4. ____ medial
5. ____ lateral
6. ____ superior
7. ____ inferior
8. ____ distal
9. ____ proximal
10. ____ bilateral
11. ____ superficial
12. ____ dorsal
13. ____ apex
14. ____ base
15. ____ inversion
16. ____ eversion
17. ____ prone
18. ____ supine
19. ____ Fowler's position
20. ____ unilateral
21. ____ recovery position
22. ____ abduction
23. ____ adduction
24. ____ extension
25. ____ flexion

a. outward movement, as in a foot twisting out
b. to move away from the body
c. movement of a joint that narrows the angle
d. directional term for both sides of the body
e. lying face down
f. turning inward
g. a reference, facing forward, palms forward
h. top of an object
i. sitting at a 45–60-degree angle
j. lying face up
k. study of the structure of an organism
l. side of a structure
m. study of function of an organism
n. away from core of the body
o. at or near the surface
p. also known as left lateral recovery position
q. a point on one side of the body
r. toward the core of the trunk of the body
s. lower than the reference point
t. movement of a joint that widens the angle
u. bottom of an object
v. to move toward the body
w. toward the midline of the body
x. back of a surface
y. point of a triangle

Integumentary System

Fill in the Blank:

1. One of the most important functions of the skin is that it __________________ us from disease.
2. The __________________ is the outermost layer of the skin.
3. Capillaries and nerve endings are found in the __________________.
4. Fat stored within the __________________ layer serves as insulation.
5. The __________________ of the skin serves as a diagnostic tool.

Muscular System

True or False: Read each statement and decide if it is true or false. Place T or F on the line before each statement.

1. _____ The ability of muscles to shorten permits movement.
2. _____ The temporal muscle is considered an accessory breathing muscle.
3. _____ The biceps, triceps, and deltoid muscles are located in the lower arm.
4. _____ The thoracic muscle divides the abdominal cavity from the chest cavity.
5. _____ The quadriceps permits extension of the leg.

Skeletal System

Matching: Match each word or term with its definition.

1. _____	appendicular skeleton	a.	includes skull, ribs, and spinal column
2. _____	axial skeleton	b.	has multiple facial bones and the cranium
3. _____	foot	c.	has a series of bones stacked on top of each other
4. _____	hand	d.	surrounds and protects the heart and lungs
5. _____	lower arm	e.	also called the breastbone
6. _____	lower leg	f.	description of the bones forming the limbs
7. _____	patella	g.	made up of the clavicle and the scapulas
8. _____	pelvic girdle	h.	the humerus
9. _____	shoulder girdle	i.	also called the forearm
10. _____	skull	j.	carpals, metacarpals, and phalanges
11. _____	spinal column	k.	supports all the weight of the body
12. _____	sternum	l.	has the longest and strongest bone in the body
13. _____	thoracic cage	m.	a bony disc that protects the inner joint
14. _____	upper arm	n.	contains the tibia and the fibula
15. _____	upper leg	o.	contains the tarsals and calcaneus

Labeling: Label each diagram in Figure 5-1 with the names of the bones shown.

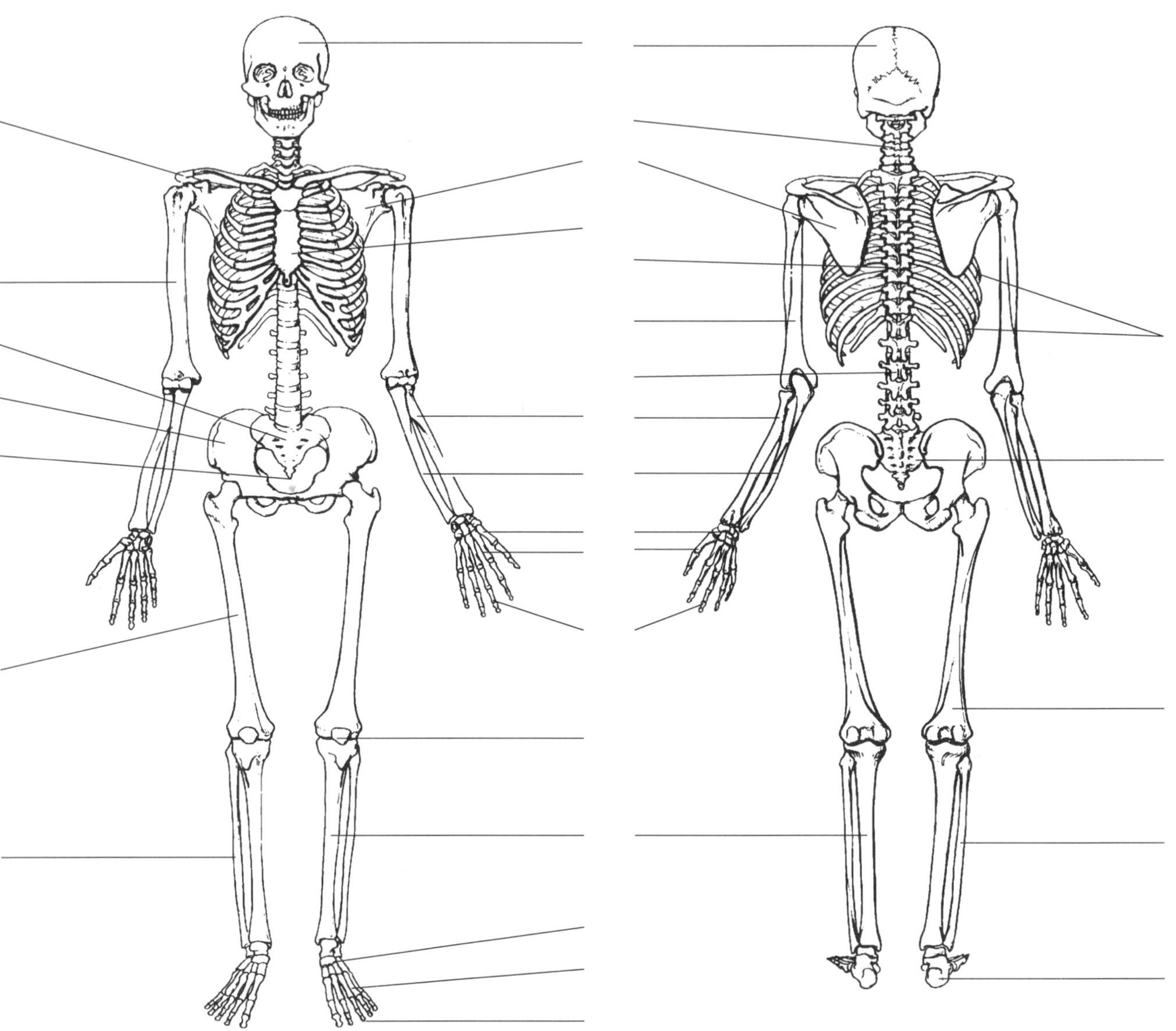

Figure 5-1

Central Nervous System

Fill in the Blank:

The central nervous system is made up of the _____________ and the ___________ ______________. It is involved in the ___________________ and ________________ of all control messages in the body. The brain consists of the _____________, the ______________, and the ____________ ______________. The brainstem consists of the _____________, _____________, and _____________. The brainstem controls life-sustaining functions such as _________________ and _____________. The "athletic brain" is called the ________________________. The "athletic brain" controls _________________ ________________. The largest area of the brain, the seat of higher thinking, is called the _________________. The brain is protected by three membranes called the ______ __________, ____________, and the __________ ____________. The brain is also protected by a fluid called ______________________ __________. The spinal cord begins at the __________ of the __________. The ___________ _____________ ____________ is made up of nerves that run from the spinal cord to take messages to the body. Automatic functions such as the heart beating are under control of the ________________ ________________ ________________.

Labeling: Label the diagram of the central nervous system in Figure 5-2.

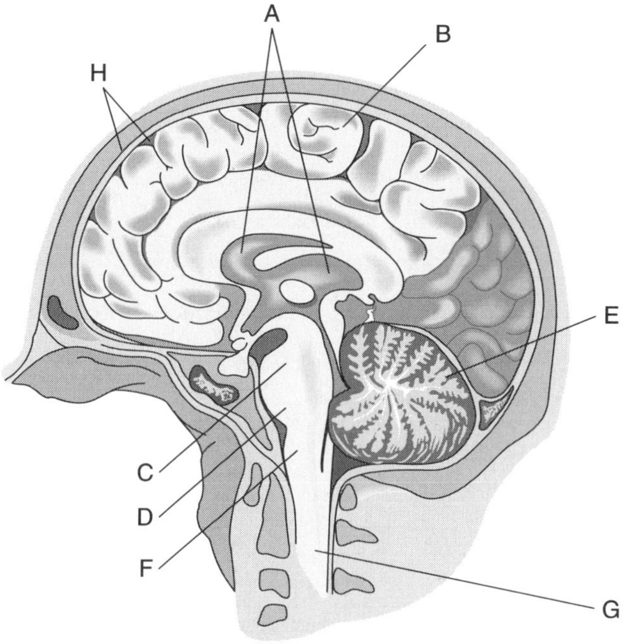

Figure 5-2

A. ______________________________

B. ______________________________

C. ______________________________

D. ______________________________

E. ______________________________

F. ______________________________

G. ______________________________

H. ______________________________

Endocrine System

Fill in the Blank:

The ____________ ________________ produces ________________, which are chemicals designed to help the nervous system maintain control of the body. The chemicals are produced by organs called ________________ and are excreted into the ____________. They then affect ________________ organs to change the way the organs function. The pancreas is relevant to the EMT-B because it produces ____________ that helps the body use ________________. Diabetics cannot produce this chemical.

Circulatory System

True or False: Read each statement and decide if it is true or false. Place T or F on the line before each statement.

1. _____ The action of blood flowing is called circulation.
2. _____ Blood vessels are unable to alter their size and distribution.
3. _____ The heart is located between the sternum and the spine.
4. _____ The heart is covered by a tough membrane called the arachnoid.
5. _____ The right side of the heart (right pump) sends blood to the systemic circuit.
6. _____ Each side of the heart has a receiving chamber called an atrium.
7. _____ The atria perform the actual work of circulating the blood to the tissues.

8. _____ Capillaries allow tissues to extract oxygen and nutrients from the blood.
9. _____ The largest artery in the body is called the vena cava.
10. _____ Vessels that return blood to the heart are called veins.

Fill in the Blank:

Beginning at the ________________ ________________, a drop of blood flows past the ________________ valve and into the right ________________. From there it passes the ________________ valve into the pulmonary ________________ and onto the lungs. Passing through the pulmonary circulation, the drop of blood returns to the left ________________ by the pulmonary ________________. Moving through the left side of the heart, the blood passes the ________________ valve into the left ________________, passes the ________________ valve and into the ________________, which is the largest artery in the body. This artery helps deliver blood to body tissues. Oxygen and nutrients are removed, and the blood returns to the right atrium via the ________________ ________________.

Labeling: Label the diagram of the heart in Figure 5-3.

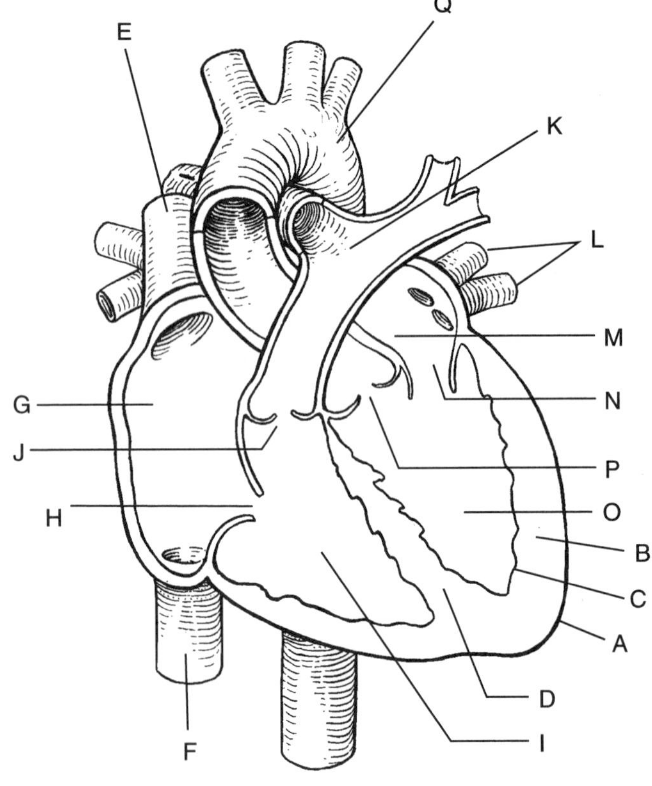

Figure 5-3

A. ______________________
B. ______________________
C. ______________________
D. ______________________
E. ______________________
F. ______________________
G. ______________________
H. ______________________
I. ______________________
J. ______________________
K. ______________________
L. ______________________
M. ______________________
N. ______________________
O. ______________________
P. ______________________
Q. ______________________

Respiratory System

Matching: Match each word or term with its definition.

1. ____ ventilation
2. ____ respiration
3. ____ upper airway
4. ____ lower airway
5. ____ trachea
6. ____ larynx
7. ____ epiglottis
8. ____ carina
9. ____ bronchus
10. ____ alveoli
11. ____ parietal pleura
12. ____ diaphragm
13. ____ visceral pleura
14. ____ bronchioles
15. ____ oropharynx

a. air sacs that permit the exchange of oxygen and carbon dioxide
b. cartilage tubes that carry air to the lungs
c. small muscular tubes connecting to the alveoli
d. point where the right and left bronchi begin
e. muscle separating the chest from the abdomen
f. protects the trachea from foreign bodies
g. section of airway visible from the mouth
h. contains the vocal cords
i. lung covering that lines the chest wall
j. exchange of gases
k. tube that connects the upper airway to the lungs
l. movement of air in and out of the lungs
m. lung covering that covers the lungs
n. purpose is to clean the outside air
o. includes the terminal bronchioles and the lungs

Labeling: Label each section of the airway on the diagram in Figure 5-4.

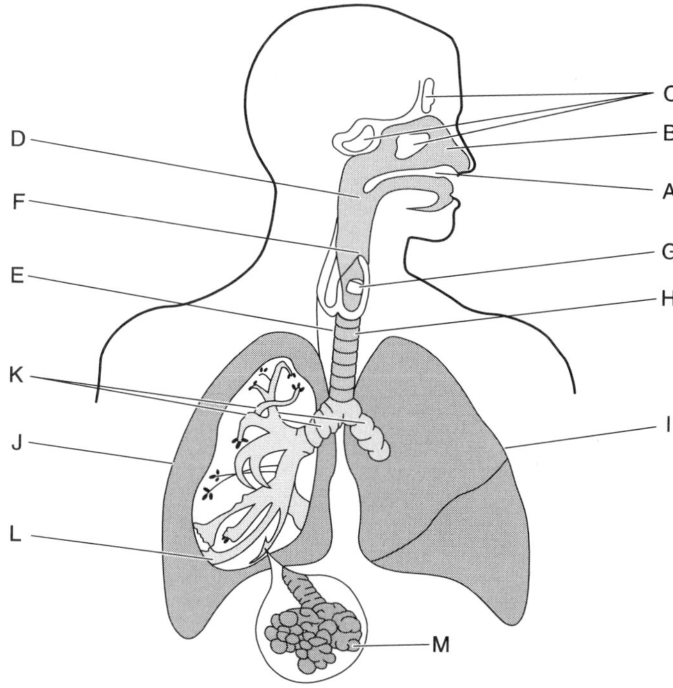

Figure 5-4

A. ____________________
B. ____________________
C. ____________________
D. ____________________
E. ____________________
F. ____________________
G. ____________________
H. ____________________
I ____________________
J. ____________________
K. ____________________
L. ____________________
M. ____________________

Digestive System

Fill in the Blank: Trace the movement of food through the body by completing the following.

The beginning of digestion takes place in the ______________. There, the teeth grind the food and allow it to be mixed with ______________, a digestive enzyme. The mass of moistened, chewed food is called a ______________ and it passes the oropharynx and into the ______________, a muscular tube connected to the stomach. There, stomach ______________ and other enzymes break the food apart. The stomach empties into the ______________ intestine where 90% of the digestion actually takes place. This intestine takes up the largest part of the abdominal cavity. Food then moves into the ______________ intestine, which terminates at the rectum. The rectum forms the feces, or waste products, which are expelled through the anus.

Completion: Complete the following table.

Organ	Type	Location	Function
liver	________	______________	detoxifies poisons
______________	hollow	______________	stores bile
pancreas	________	center	______________________
appendix	________	______________	unknown
______________	solid	retroperitoneal	______________________

Labeling: Label the diagram of the digestive system in Figure 5-5.

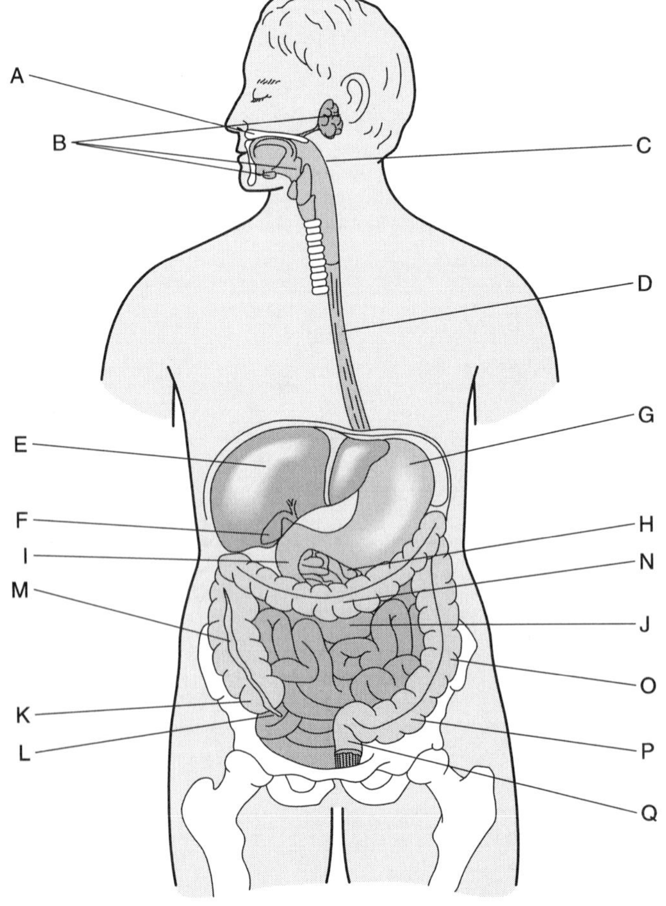

Figure 5-5

A. ______________________________

B. ______________________________

C. ______________________________

D. ______________________________

E. ______________________________

F. ______________________________

G. ______________________________

H. ______________________________

I. ______________________________

J. ______________________________

K. ______________________________

L. ______________________________

M. ______________________________

N. ______________________________

O. ______________________________

P. ______________________________

Q. ______________________________

Reproductive System

Matching: Match each word or term with its definition.

1. ____	testes	a.	male and female organs of reproduction
2. ____	scrotum	b.	monthly flow resulting if fertilization doesn't occur
3. ____	penis	c.	produces female sex hormones
4. ____	sperm	d.	conduit for sperm or urine
5. ____	prostate	e.	gland that produces fluid to transport sperm
6. ____	ovary	f.	sac enclosing the testes
7. ____	fallopian tube	g.	responsible for fertilization of the egg
8. ____	uterus	h.	male gonad
9. ____	menstruation	i.	organ where a fetus grows and matures
10. ____	vagina	j.	allows for delivery of the baby
11. ____	gonads	k.	allows the egg to go from the ovary to the uterus

Labeling: Label the diagrams of the male and female reproductive systems in Figures 5-6a and 5-6b.

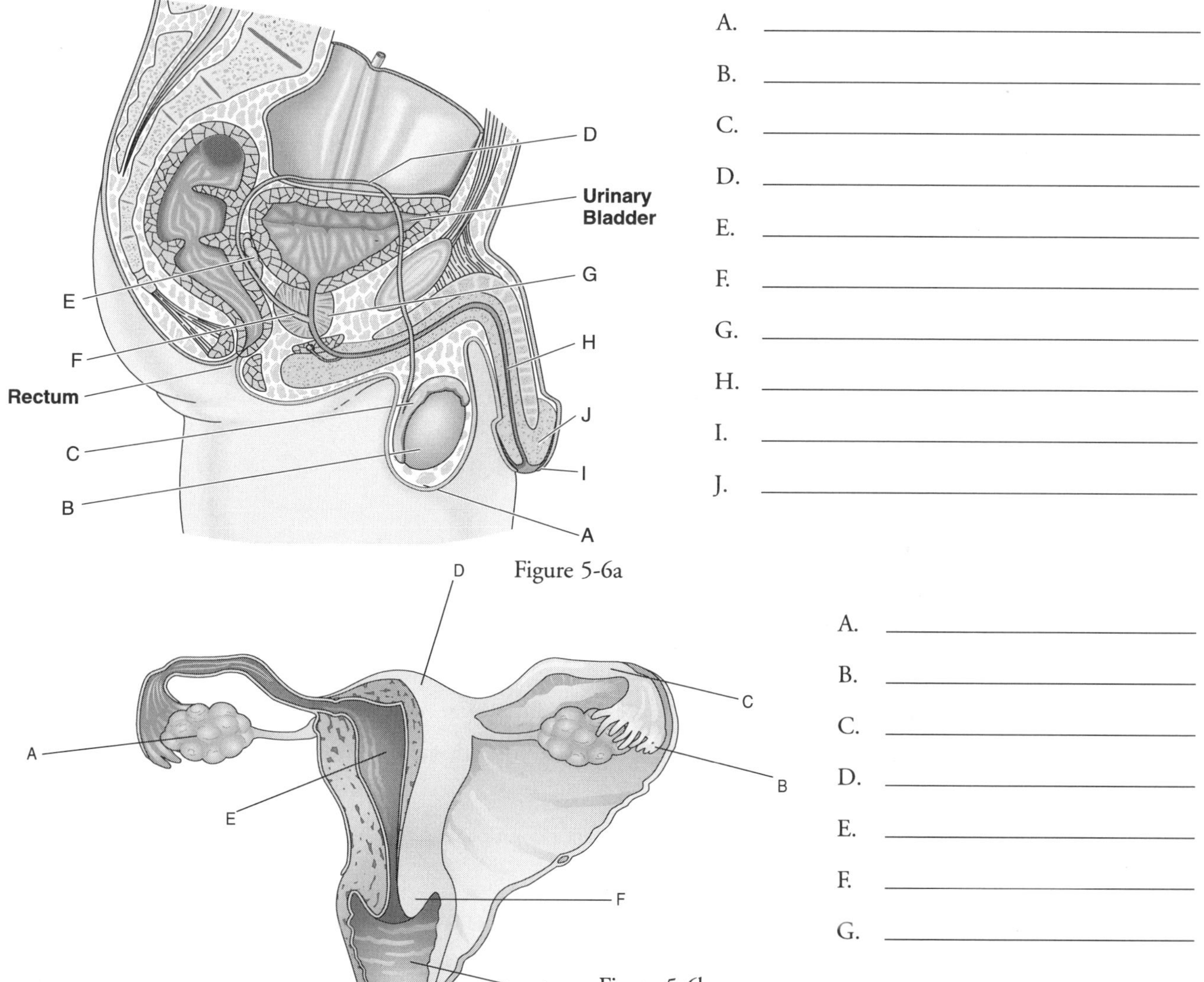

Figure 5-6a

A. ______________________

B. ______________________

C. ______________________

D. ______________________

E. ______________________

F. ______________________

G. ______________________

H. ______________________

I. ______________________

J. ______________________

Figure 5-6b

A. ______________________

B. ______________________

C. ______________________

D. ______________________

E. ______________________

F. ______________________

G. ______________________

CHAPTER 6
Infection Control

Whenever an EMT-B approaches a sick or injured patient, there is a danger of contracting an infectious disease. For this reason, EMT-Bs must learn disease prevention and infection control.

Word Scramble: Unscramble the following words from the Key Terms in Chapter 6 of the textbook.

1. tiumnonmziia ______________________
2. rrracie ______________________
3. aprxhpylios ______________________
4. sinomisntsor ______________________
5. gtacnosuio ______________________
6. oopcmmsciromunum ______________________
7. biantody ______________________
8. ocrimmsinorga ______________________
9. trocve ______________________
10. zihaabrdo ______________________

Listing:

A. List five examples of common illnesses and give their mode of transmission.

1.
2.
3.
4.
5.

B. Give two examples of standards designed to protect EMTs from disease.

1.
2.

True or False: Read each statement and decide if it is true or false. Place T or F on the line before each statement.

1. ____ EMTs are at risk from infectious diseases only when the patient is bleeding.
2. ____ EMTs can expose patients to infectious diseases.
3. ____ An infection is caused by microscopic living creatures.
4. ____ Transmission of disease between people occurs only by direct contact.
5. ____ For disease to occur, the strength of the disease must overcome the host's defenses.
6. ____ All infectious diseases have immunizations.
7. ____ The EMT must take Standard Precautions when caring for a patient.
8. ____ There are no barrier devices available for the eyes.
9. ____ All waste generated on a patient care scene is considered a biohazard.
10. ____ EMTs can become carriers of disease while not becoming sick themselves.

Definitions: Write the definitions of the following terms.

safety officer ______________________________

biohazard ______________________________

personal protective equipment ______________________________

immunocompromised ______________________________

infection control manual ______________________________

risk profile ______________________________

Identification: Check the appropriate behaviors in preventing infection.

_____ Ongoing health assessment of the EMT.

_____ Putting on gloves, gown, and mask before any patient encounter, and then removing what is unnecessary.

_____ Carrying spare gloves for use with multiple patients.

_____ Washing hands only if gloves are unavailable or ripped.

_____ Using goggles or safety glasses to protect the eyes.

_____ Putting on a mask only if you are close to a patient.

_____ Using a gown for imminent childbirth.

_____ Using latex gloves for handling body fluids, and vinyl gloves for patient contact.

Fill in the Blank: Complete the following sentences that describe putting on and removing personal protective equipment.

The EMT should first put on ____________ and ____________ protection. She should then put on the ____________ if it is necessary. Assistance may be needed in ____________ the ____________ in back. Put the ____________ on last. To remove the PPE, the EMT should go in ____________ order. Remove the ____________. Then reach back and ____________ or ____________ the ties of the ____________ Turn it inside out and roll it into a ball. Last remove the ____________ and ____________ protection. Finally, ____________ your hands.

Matching: Match each word or term with its definition.

1. ____ Bloodborne Pathogens Rule
2. ____ Centers for Disease Control and Prevention
3. ____ high-level disinfection
4. ____ intermediate-level disinfection
5. ____ infection control manual
6. ____ OSHA
7. ____ National Fire Protection Association
8. ____ sterilization
9. ____ Ryan White Law
10. ____ risk management

a. set of rules for employers regarding infection control practices
b. wiping down the surface with an EPA-registered germicide or bleach solution
c. document that lists infection prevention procedures
d. requirement of hospitals to notify an EMS agency of a potential exposure to infectious disease
e. actions geared toward protection from infectious disease
f. federal organization that monitors transmission of infection
g. federal organization that sets association standards for preventing on-the-job illness or injury
h. required for equipment that touches a patient's mucous membranes
i. organization that sets requirements for firefighters
j. thorough cleaning so that all microorganisms are removed

Identification: Place a checkmark in front of each of the following diseases that have an immunization available.

_____ AIDS _____ rubella

_____ tuberculosis _____ tetanus

_____ hepatitis B _____ measles

Identification: State whether each of the following is an airborne, contact, vehicle, or vector-borne transmission by writing the correct word on the line in front.

1. ____________________ An EMT with a cold sneezes near another person who inhales the droplets.
2. ____________________ A paramedic eats food contaminated with salmonella.
3. ____________________ A paramedic accidentally sticks herself with a bloody needle.
4. ____________________ An EMT drinks contaminated water and develops diarrhea.
5. ____________________ A tick bites a child who becomes sick.
6. ____________________ A nurse develops a tear in her glove and blood enters an open cut.
7. ____________________ The paramedic touches dried blood on a stretcher and becomes ill.
8. ____________________ A patient coughs near the EMT who has not yet donned a mask.

Short Answer: Read each question. Think about the information presented in your text, and then answer each question with one or two sentences.

1. Explain how handwashing is the single most important act in preventing the spread of infectious diseases.

2. List the occasions when the EMT may use waterless cleansers.

3. After using a waterless cleanser, when should the EMT perform hand washing with soap and water?

Critical Thinking: Read the following case study and then answer the questions.

Jess and Stephanie responded to a "man injured" while he was cutting shrubbery. Upon their arrival, they put on their gloves and proceeded to assess their patient, Mr. Ricci. He was alert but scared and bleeding profusely from arm and hand injuries caused by electric shrub shears. Stephanie proceeded to care for the bleeding while Jess ensured that the shears were turned off and moved out of the way. While Stephanie and Jess assisted Mr. Ricci to the ambulance, Jess noticed that her glove had a jagged rip and the skin underneath was scraped.

1. What should Jess do now?

2. How can Jess accomplish this?

3. What should she do next?

4. Jess has been directed to see a physician while at the emergency department. Why is this necessary?

Chapter 6 Skill Sheet

Student Name ________________________________ Date ________________

Skill 6-1: Hand Washing

Equipment Needed:

1. Soap
2. Water
3. Hand brush

Yes: ❑ Reteach: ❑ Return: ❑ Instructor initials: ________

Step 1: Remove any rings, watch, or other jewelry that could trap contaminations.

Yes: ❑ Reteach: ❑ Return: ❑ Instructor initials: ________

Step 2: Turn on the water and adjust it to a comfortable temperature. The water should flow freely.

Yes: ❑ Reteach: ❑ Return: ❑ Instructor initials: ________

Step 3: Liberally apply the soap. Scrub vigorously, rubbing the hands together to create friction. Particular attention should be paid to the space in between the fingers and the area under the nails. Scrub for at least one minute.

Yes: ❑ Reteach: ❑ Return: ❑ Instructor initials: ________

Step 4: Rinse the hands, allowing the contaminated water to run off the elbow.

Yes: ❑ Reteach: ❑ Return: ❑ Instructor initials: ________

Step 5: Turn off the faucet with a clean towel. Dry the hands with a clean towel, starting at the fingers and working toward the elbow.

Yes: ❑ Reteach: ❑ Return: ❑ Instructor initials: ________

Chapter 6 Skill Sheet

Student Name ______________________ Date ____________

Skill 6-2A: Donning Personal Protective Equipment (PPE)

Equipment Needed:

1. Mask
2. Goggles
3. Gown
4. Nonsterile examination gloves (EMTs with latex sensitivity should wear vinyl gloves)

Yes: ❑ Reteach: ❑ Return: ❑ Instructor initials: ________

Step 1: Grasp the top ties of the mask and position the metal strip in the mask over the bridge of the nose.

Yes: ❑ Reteach: ❑ Return: ❑ Instructor initials: ________

Step 2: Pull the elastic straps over the head.

Yes: ❑ Reteach: ❑ Return: ❑ Instructor initials: ________

Step 3: Grasp and pinch the metal strip around the bridge of the nose.

Yes: ❑ Reteach: ❑ Return: ❑ Instructor initials: ________

Step 4: Apply eye protection.

Yes: ❑ Reteach: ❑ Return: ❑ Instructor initials: ________

Step 5: Hold the gown up by the collar with the inside facing you.

Yes: ❑ Reteach: ❑ Return: ❑ Instructor initials: ________

(continues)

Chapter 6 Skill Sheet

Skill 6-2A: *Continued*

Step 6: Place one arm then the other into the gown.

Yes: ❑ Reteach: ❑ Return: ❑ Instructor initials: ________

Step 7: Reach around behind your neck and tie the neck ties snugly.

Yes: ❑ Reteach: ❑ Return: ❑ Instructor initials: ________

Step 8: Pull on properly sized examination gloves. Each glove's collar should be over the sleeve of the gown.

Yes: ❑ Reteach: ❑ Return: ❑ Instructor initials: ________

Chapter 6 Skill Sheet

Student Name ______________________ Date ____________

Skill 6-2B: Removing Personal Protective Equipment (PPE)

Step 1: After removal of contaminated gloves, the EMT should untie (or break if a paper gown) the waist and neck ties of the gown. If the gown is grossly contaminated, the EMT should ask a partner to do this to avoid contamination of her ungloved hands.

Yes: ❑ Reteach: ❑ Return: ❑ Instructor initials: ________

Step 2: With the left hand, grasp the right neckline of the gown, as close to the shoulder as possible without contamination, and pull the gown off the front of the body.

Yes: ❑ Reteach: ❑ Return: ❑ Instructor initials: ________

Step 3: As the gown is pulled forward, it should be removed from the right arm.

Yes: ❑ Reteach: ❑ Return: ❑ Instructor initials: ________

Step 4: The ungloved right hand can then grasp the uncontaminated inner surface of the gown and pull it off the left arm.

Yes: ❑ Reteach: ❑ Return: ❑ Instructor initials: ________

Step 5: Careful to touch only the uncontaminated inner surface of the gown, the EMT should roll the gown up and dispose of it in the appropriate hazardous waste container.

Yes: ❑ Reteach: ❑ Return: ❑ Instructor initials: ________

Step 6: Reaching behind the head, the EMT should untie, or tear, the ties from the mask.

Yes: ❑ Reteach: ❑ Return: ❑ Instructor initials: ________

Step 7: The mask should be held by the uncontaminated ties and pulled away from the face.

Yes: ❑ Reteach: ❑ Return: ❑ Instructor initials: ________

Step 8: The contaminated mask should be disposed of in the proper hazardous waste container.

Yes: ❑ Reteach: ❑ Return: ❑ Instructor initials: ________

Chapter 6 Skill Sheet

Student Name ______________________________ Date ________________

Skill 6-3A: Donning Gloves

Equipment Needed:

Nonsterile examination gloves

Yes: ❑ Reteach: ❑ Return: ❑ Instructor initials: ________

Step 1: Choose an appropriate size and type of glove for the task at hand. Arrange one glove so that the thumb is aligned with the thumb of the hand it is intended to go on.

Yes: ❑ Reteach: ❑ Return: ❑ Instructor initials: ________

Step 2: Grasp the front of the cuff with one hand, while sliding the other hand into the glove. Be sure to place each finger within the appropriate finger section. Pull at the cuff to ensure that the glove is completely applied to the hand.

Yes: ❑ Reteach: ❑ Return: ❑ Instructor initials: ________

Step 3: Repeat the process for the other hand.

Yes: ❑ Reteach: ❑ Return: ❑ Instructor initials: ________

Chapter 6 Skill Sheet

Student Name ______________________ Date ____________

Skill 6-3B: Removing Gloves

Equipment Needed:

Approved biohazard container

Yes: ❑ Reteach: ❑ Return: ❑ Instructor initials: ________

Step 1: Grasp the palm of the left glove with the gloved right hand.

Yes: ❑ Reteach: ❑ Return: ❑ Instructor initials: ________

Step 2: Pull the left glove toward the fingertips. The glove should turn inside out as it is removed.

Yes: ❑ Reteach: ❑ Return: ❑ Instructor initials: ________

Step 3: Hold the removed glove in the still gloved right hand. Place two fingers of the ungloved left hand under the cuff of the right glove, carefully avoiding any contaminated areas. Pull the right glove toward the fingertips, turning it inside out as it is removed. The soiled left glove should remain in the palm of the right glove as it is removed.

Yes: ❑ Reteach: ❑ Return: ❑ Instructor initials: ________

Step 4: Dispose of the gloves in an approved biohazard container. Wash hands thoroughly.

Yes: ❑ Reteach: ❑ Return: ❑ Instructor initials: ________

CHAPTER 7
Basic Airway Control

The human body needs oxygen in order for cells to produce energy. Oxygen gets into the body by first moving through the airway. Whenever a patient cannot keep her airway open, the EMT must keep it open.

Matching: Match each word or term with its definition.

1. _____	esophagus	a.	upper jawbone
2. _____	mandible	b.	swings up to protect the nasal cavity
3. _____	maxilla	c.	most common cause of airway obstruction
4. _____	larynx	d.	protects the top of the lower airway
5. _____	nostrils	e.	pillars of fragile soft tissues in the throat
6. _____	pharynx	f.	food passageway
7. _____	uvula	g.	voice box
8. _____	tonsils	h.	lower jawbone
9. _____	tongue	i.	back of throat where oral and nasal cavities meet
10. _____	epiglottis	j.	openings to the nose from outside

Definitions: Write the definitions of the following terms.

ventilation ______________________________

apnea ______________________________

cyanosis ______________________________

epiglottis ______________________________

nasal flaring ______________________________

sputum ______________________________

sublingual ______________________________

gag reflex ______________________________

occlusion ______________________________

Yankauer tip ______________________________

Identification: Place a checkmark in front of each word or phrase that is a sign or symptom of an obstructed or collapsed airway.

_____ apnea	_____ cough	_____ conjunctiva
_____ cyanosis	_____ snoring	_____ uvula
_____ breathlessness	_____ intact dentures	_____ sneezing

Ordering: Place the following steps to opening an airway of a noninjured patient in the correct order. Put a numeral 1 before the first step, 2 before the next, and so on.

_____ Maintain open airway during entire call

_____ Avoid pressure on underside of the jaw

_____ Kneel at the level of the head

_____ Push down on the forehead and lift up on the chin

_____ Place the palm of one hand on the forehead and the fingertips on the jaw

Identification: Each of the following patients is in need of an airway assistive device, either an oropharyngeal airway (OPA) or a nasopharyngeal airway (NPA). Read each scenario and then write the name of the correct device on the line in front of each one.

1. ____________________ The patient gagged when she was orally suctioned
2. ____________________ An unconscious patient
3. ____________________ A patient having a seizure who has clenched her teeth
4. ____________________ The patient was bleeding profusely from her nose
5. ____________________ There was no gag reflex with a fingersweep
6. ____________________ The patient's wife states that he has a history of nasal bleeding
7. ____________________ The patient has a large amount of soft palate damage

Correcting: Each of the following sentences is false. Rewrite it as a correct statement.

1. Suctioning removes just fluids.
2. Suction, secure, open, and assess the airway.
3. Suction as deeply as the catheter will go.
4. Adequate suctioning will take 20–30 seconds.
5. Apply suction while advancing the catheter.
6. Use a French catheter to suction blood.
7. Yankauer catheters are best used for suctioning a tracheostomy.
8. Measure the depth of suctioning from the tip of the nose to the corner of the mouth.
9. Change suction catheters between each suction attempt.
10. It is not necessary to wear gloves when suctioning.

Critical Thinking: Read the following case study and then answer the questions.

Tania and Geoff are called to Castings Manufacturing Co. for a worker found unconscious next to his machine. The worker, John Wojtiak, is a 56-year-old man who has worked at the plant for 20 years. None of his coworkers heard or saw what happened.

1. What essential pieces of equipment must the EMTs bring to John's side?

2. What must Tania and Geoff do before using that equipment?

Upon arriving at Mr. Wojtiak's side, the EMTs find him lying on his back, snoring. They put on their PPE and begin to care for him.

3. What two signs point to a need to open the airway?

4. What method should Geoff choose to open the airway? Why?

5. What should be done next for the airway?

6. What airway assistive device should Tania place?

Following initial assessment and care, Mr. Wojtiak is placed on a backboard and a stretcher for transport to the hospital. Geoff provides care during the trip.

7. What important function must Geoff monitor and care for during the trip to the hospital? Why?

Chapter 7 Skill Sheet

Student Name ______________________________ Date ________________

Skill 7-1: Head-Tilt, Chin-Lift

Equipment Needed:

1. Gloves
2. Goggles
3. Mask

Yes: ❑ Reteach: ❑ Return: ❑ Instructor initials: ________

Step 1: After donning the appropriate PPE, the EMT should position himself at the side of the patient's head.

Yes: ❑ Reteach: ❑ Return: ❑ Instructor initials: ________

Step 2: The palm of one hand should be placed on the patient's forehead, and the fingertips of the other hand on the patient's jaw.

Yes: ❑ Reteach: ❑ Return: ❑ Instructor initials: ________

Step 3: The patient's head is tilted back using a firm pressure on the forehead. The jaw is then gently lifted up to pull the tongue off the back of the throat. Care should be taken not to push backward on the jaw, as this will only force the patient's mouth closed.

Yes: ❑ Reteach: ❑ Return: ❑ Instructor initials: ________

Chapter 7 Skill Sheet

Student Name ______________________________ Date ________________

Skill 7-2: Jaw Thrust Maneuver

Equipment Needed:

1. Gloves
2. Goggles
3. Mask

Yes: ❑ Reteach: ❑ Return: ❑ Instructor initials: ________

Step 1: After donning the appropriate PPE, the EMT should position himself above the patient's head.

Yes: ❑ Reteach: ❑ Return: ❑ Instructor initials: ________

Step 2: The EMT should place his middle and index fingers on the angles of the patient's jaw and his thumbs on the cheekbones.

Yes: ❑ Reteach: ❑ Return: ❑ Instructor initials: ________

Step 3: The middle and index fingers lift the jaw and the tongue up off of the back of the throat while avoiding any movement of the neck.

Yes: ❑ Reteach: ❑ Return: ❑ Instructor initials: ________

Chapter 7 Skill Sheet

Student Name ______________________________ Date ________________

Skill 7-3: Suctioning the Airway

Equipment Needed:

1. Gloves
2. Goggles
3. Mask
4. Suction device (electric or mechanical)
5. Tubing
6. Catheter
7. Water

Yes: ❑ Reteach: ❑ Return: ❑ Instructor initials: ________

Step 1: One EMT opens and assesses the airway, using the technique appropriate to the patient's situation.

Yes: ❑ Reteach: ❑ Return: ❑ Instructor initials: ________

Step 2: Another EMT removes the rigid suction tip from its protective covering, attaches the tip to the tubing, and then the tubing to the intake of the suction machine. Once the equipment is assembled, the EMT tests the machine's suction.

Yes: ❑ Reteach: ❑ Return: ❑ Instructor initials: ________

Step 3: The distance from the opening of the mouth to the angle of the jaw should be measured as an estimate of the length of the suction tip.

Yes: ❑ Reteach: ❑ Return: ❑ Instructor initials: ________

Step 4: The EMT should use the cross-fingered technique to open the patient's mouth. Start by crossing the thumb under the index finger and placing the thumb against the lower teeth and the index finger against the upper teeth.

Yes: ❑ Reteach: ❑ Return: ❑ Instructor initials: ________

Step 5: The rigid suction tip is then inserted to the depth of the measurement. A thumb can be placed over the whistle port on the tip to generate suction. Suction should be applied while the tip is being removed from the mouth, and should never be allowed to remain constant for more than 15 seconds. The patient should then be reassessed, oxygen reapplied, and the procedure repeated as necessary.

Yes: ❑ Reteach: ❑ Return: ❑ Instructor initials: ________

Chapter 7 Skill Sheet

Student Name ______________________ Date ____________

Skill 7-4: Oropharyngeal Airway Insertion

Equipment Needed:

1. Gloves
2. Goggles
3. Mask
4. Assortment of oral airways

Yes: ❑ Reteach: ❑ Return: ❑ Instructor initials: ________

Step 1: The EMT must manually open the airway, using the technique appropriate to the patient's condition. The patient's airway should be suctioned as needed.

Yes: ❑ Reteach: ❑ Return: ❑ Instructor initials: ________

Step 2: The EMT then chooses an oral airway that fits the patient. The length of the oral airway should match the distance from the angle of the jaw to the opening of the mouth.

Yes: ❑ Reteach: ❑ Return: ❑ Instructor initials: ________

Step 3: Using the cross-fingered technique, the EMT should open the patient's mouth. The proper size airway should be initially guided into the patient's mouth with the curvature facing downward, toward the jaw, to about midway.

Yes: ❑ Reteach: ❑ Return: ❑ Instructor initials: ________

Step 4: The EMT then rotates the oral airway 180 degrees so that the airway follows the curvature of the hard palate.

Yes: ❑ Reteach: ❑ Return: ❑ Instructor initials: ________

Step 5: Alternatively, the EMT can use a tongue depressor to press the tongue downward and forward. Then an oral airway may be inserted directly into the oral cavity, following the curve of the hard palate.

Yes: ❑ Reteach: ❑ Return: ❑ Instructor initials: ________

Step 6: The OPA should rest with the flange against the patient's lips.

Yes: ❑ Reteach: ❑ Return: ❑ Instructor initials: ________

Chapter 7 Skill Sheet

Student Name ______________________________ Date ________________

Skill 7-5: Nasopharyngeal Airway Insertion

Equipment Needed:

1. Gloves
2. Goggles
3. Mask
4. Assortment of nasal airways
5. Water-soluble lubricant

Yes: ❑ Reteach: ❑ Return: ❑ Instructor initials: ________

Step 1: The EMT first examines the nostril opening to determine an appropriate size of nasal airway that will be needed.

Yes: ❑ Reteach: ❑ Return: ❑ Instructor initials: ________

Step 2: The properly sized nasal airway will reach from the nostril to the tip of the earlobe.

Yes: ❑ Reteach: ❑ Return: ❑ Instructor initials: ________

Step 3: The nasal airway should be generously lubricated with a water-soluble lubricant to ease placement.

Yes: ❑ Reteach: ❑ Return: ❑ Instructor initials: ________

Step 4: The lubricated nasal airway should be placed into the nostril with the bevel facing the nasal septum (middle of the nose).

Yes: ❑ Reteach: ❑ Return: ❑ Instructor initials: ________

Step 5: A gentle corkscrewing action, back and forth, as the EMT gently pushes straight backward usually allows the nasal airway to be placed.

Yes: ❑ Reteach: ❑ Return: ❑ Instructor initials: ________

Step 6: If resistance is met, then the nasal airway should be withdrawn and insertion into the other nostril attempted.

Yes: ❑ Reteach: ❑ Return: ❑ Instructor initials: ________

NREMT Skill Sheet

Airway, Oxygen and Ventilation Skills: Upper Airway Adjuncts and Suction

Start Time: ______________________

Stop Time: ______________________ **Date:** ______________

Candidate's Name: ______________________________________

Evaluator's Name: ______________________________________

OROPHARYNGEAL AIRWAY	Points Possible	Points Awarded
Takes, or verbalizes, body substance isolation precautions	1	
Selects appropriately sized airway	1	
Measures airway	1	
Inserts airway without pushing the tongue posteriorly	1	
Note: The examiner must advise the candidate that the patient is gagging and becoming conscious.		
Removes the oropharyngeal airway	1	

SUCTION

Note: The examiner must advise the candidate to suction the patient's airway.		
Turns on/prepares suction device	1	
Assures presence of mechanical suction	1	
Inserts the suction tip without suction	1	
Applies suction to the oropharynx/nasopharynx	1	

NASOPHARYNGEAL AIRWAY

Note: The examiner must advise the candidate to insert a nasopharyngeal airway.		
Selects appropriately sized airway	1	
Measures airway	1	
Verbalizes lubrication of the nasal airway	1	
Fully inserts the airway with the bevel facing toward the septum	1	
Total:	13	

Critical Criteria

_______ Did not take, or verbalize, body substance isolation precautions

_______ Did not obtain a patent airway with the oropharyngeal airway

_______ Did not obtain a patent airway with the nasopharyngeal airway

_______ Did not demonstrate an acceptable suction technique

CHAPTER 8
Respiratory Support

The public has come to expect that EMTs are the experts in the techniques of respiratory support.

Matching: Match each word or term with its definition.

1. _____ hypoxia	a. posture of those in respiratory distress
2. _____ contraindication	b. the feeling of difficulty breathing
3. _____ air hunger	c. a lung disease
4. _____ apnea	d. reasons to do something
5. _____ dentures	e. allows for oxygen flow in liters per minute
6. _____ hypoventilation	f. false teeth
7. _____ dyspnea	g. insufficient body stores of oxygen
8. _____ tripod position	h. device that measures oxygen on red cells
9. _____ stoma	i. to feel with one's hands
10. _____ emphysema	j. breathing faster than normal
11. _____ indication	k. bypassing warming and filtering to get air in
12. _____ regulator	l. breathing slower or ineffectively
13. _____ tachypnea	m. reasons not to do something
14. _____ palpate	n. lack of breathing
15. _____ pulse oximeter	o. hole created after laryngectomy

Identification: Read the definitions. Write the correct word or terms on the line.

1. ________________________ muscles in the neck and chest that aid in breathing
2. ________________________ to listen
3. ________________________ compresses the esophagus
4. ________________________ muscles between the ribs
5. ________________________ instillation of moisture
6. ________________________ area that does not participate in gas exchange
7. ________________________ a device placed in nose, delivers 25–44% oxygen
8. ________________________ device that delivers nearly 100% oxygen
9. ________________________ exhaling past partially closed lips when in distress
10. ________________________ surgical hole to enable effective ventilation

Identification: Place a checkmark in front of each word or phrase that is a sign or symptom of respiratory distress.

___ seesaw breathing	___ cricoid pressure	___ tripod
___ air hunger	___ apex	___ uvula
___ pursed lip breathing	___ accessory muscle use	___ sneezing

Short Answer: Read each question. Think about the information presented in your text, and then answer each question with one or two sentences.

1. How much oxygen is normally contained in air?

2. What is ventilation?

3. What is oxygenation?

4. Can ventilation occur without oxygenation? Describe.

Identification: For each description, write the name of the device.

1. ______________________ clear, plastic dome-shaped device, with an air cushion to provide a seal; may have a filter and an oxygen inlet port
2. ______________________ originated from an anesthesia bag; is self-inflating
3. ______________________ a device that runs on oxygen; has a trigger to operate and can be used by one person
4. ______________________ a clear mask with an oxygen reservoir; delivers high concentration oxygen when set at 10 lpm or greater
5. ______________________ a small "mask" that fits over a stoma
6. ______________________ blue and corrugated, designed for use on transports of greater than an hour
7. ______________________ oxygen is delivered via prongs to the nose

Short Answer: Explain the possible consequences of failing to follow each of these safety tips regarding the use of oxygen.

1. Smoking near oxygen tanks.

2. Allowing petroleum products near tanks or fittings.

3. Storing oxygen in extreme temperatures.

4. Using a modified regulator from another gas cylinder.

5. Leaving an oxygen tank unattended.

6. Placing a portable oxygen tank standing up.

Critical Thinking: Read the following case study and then answer the questions.

Chris and Danny had just arrived back at the station when they were called to a home several blocks away. The caller had stated that her father was "having a little difficulty breathing." When they entered the man's room, Danny hung back for a second and watched the man. Chris began interviewing the daughter.

1. What is Danny looking for?

2. What information will Chris miss by interviewing the daughter?

The father, Mr. Allen, was sitting bolt upright with his hands on his knees. When he tried to speak to his daughter, he could manage only one word per breath. Danny noted that when Mr. Allen exhaled, he blew air out as if he was blowing out a candle.

3. What are the terms used to describe the observations made by Danny?

4. What assessments should Danny and Chris make next?

Chris used his stethoscope to listen to Mr. Allen's lungs. He heard air moving in and out on both sides, but it was accompanied by high-pitched wheezing. He placed a pulse oximeter on Mr. Allen's finger while Danny set up an oxygen mask.

5. What is the term for listening with a stethoscope?

6. What do the EMTs know about Mr. Allen's breathing and lung status based on their exam so far?

Danny placed a non-rebreather mask with 10 lpm oxygen on Mr. Allen and called dispatch to request a paramedic to the scene.

7. What percentage of oxygen is delivered by a non-rebreather mask at 10 lpm?

8. What should be done next for the airway?

9. What airway assistive device should Danny place on Mr. Allen?

Chapter 8 Skill Sheet

Student Name ______________________________ Date ________________

Skill 8-1: Oxygen Tank Assembly

Equipment Needed:

1. Oxygen tank
2. Regulator

Yes: ❑ Reteach: ❑ Return: ❑ Instructor initials: ________

Step 1: The EMT should confirm that the tank at hand contains oxygen. These tanks are green in color. They have pins that match to the oxygen regulator only for safety.

Yes: ❑ Reteach: ❑ Return: ❑ Instructor initials: ________

Step 2: The EMT compares the oxygen regulator's pins with the contacts on the oxygen bottle's stem. Again, by convention, oxygen regulators have a specific pin configuration that fits only oxygen bottles.

Yes: ❑ Reteach: ❑ Return: ❑ Instructor initials: ________

Step 3: Using an oxygen wrench, the EMT should quickly open and close the oxygen tank by turning the device at the top of the tank counterclockwise, then again clockwise. This procedure, called "cracking the tank," blows out any dirt and dust in the outlet.

Yes: ❑ Reteach: ❑ Return: ❑ Instructor initials: ________

Step 4: The EMT should then mate the regulator to the oxygen tank, being sure to tightly seal the regulator. Often a plastic washer is needed for an airtight fit.

Yes: ❑ Reteach: ❑ Return: ❑ Instructor initials: ________

Step 5: The oxygen tank may now be safely opened by again turning the device at the top of the tank counterclockwise as far as it allows, then back one-quarter turn. The pressure within the tank should be noted at this time.

Yes: ❑ Reteach: ❑ Return: ❑ Instructor initials: ________

Step 6: To adjust the liter flow rate, the EMT can turn the flow adjusting knob on the regulator in a counterclockwise motion until the desired liter flow appears.

Yes: ❑ Reteach: ❑ Return: ❑ Instructor initials: ________

Chapter 8 Skill Sheet

Student Name ______________________ Date ____________

Skill 8-2: Application of a Non-Rebreather Mask

Equipment Needed:

1. Oxygen tank and regulator
2. Non-rebreather mask
3. Gloves

Yes: ❑ Reteach: ❑ Return: ❑ Instructor initials: ________

Step 1: First, the EMT must ensure that the oxygen tank and oxygen regulator are correctly assembled. The oxygen tank should have sufficient pressure to provide continuous oxygen flow.

Yes: ❑ Reteach: ❑ Return: ❑ Instructor initials: ________

Step 2: Then the EMT should choose the correct oxygen administration device. A non-rebreather mask is used when high concentrations of oxygen are desired.

Yes: ❑ Reteach: ❑ Return: ❑ Instructor initials: ________

Step 3: To use the non-rebreather mask, the EMT must attach the oxygen tubing to the regulator and turn on the regulator. The regulator should never be turned below 6 lpm.

Yes: ❑ Reteach: ❑ Return: ❑ Instructor initials: ________

Step 4: The EMT then places his thumbs over the valve between the bag and the mask, permitting the bag to fill completely.

Yes: ❑ Reteach: ❑ Return: ❑ Instructor initials: ________

Step 5: Grasping the mask in one hand and the elastic band in the other, the EMT would seat the mask firmly on the bridge of the nose and drape the elastic band around the head. The EMT should pinch the metal strap around the nose.

Yes: ❑ Reteach: ❑ Return: ❑ Instructor initials: ________

Step 6: The EMT then adjusts the liter flow to ensure that the oxygen bag is always at least one-half full.

Yes: ❑ Reteach: ❑ Return: ❑ Instructor initials: ________

Chapter 8 Skill Sheet

Student Name ________________________________ Date ________________

Skill 8-3: Application of a Nasal Cannula

Equipment Needed:

1. Oxygen tank and regulator
2. Nasal cannula
3. Gloves

Yes: ❑ Reteach: ❑ Return: ❑ Instructor initials: ________

Step 1: First, the EMT must ensure that the oxygen tank and oxygen regulator are correctly assembled. The oxygen tank should have sufficient pressure to provide continuous oxygen flow.

Yes: ❑ Reteach: ❑ Return: ❑ Instructor initials: ________

Step 2: Then the EMT should choose the correct oxygen administration device. A nasal cannula is used when the patient can tolerate the non-rebreather oxygen mask, or when low concentrations of oxygen are desired.

Yes: ❑ Reteach: ❑ Return: ❑ Instructor initials: ________

Step 3: To use the nasal cannula, the EMT must attach the oxygen tubing to the regulator and turn on the regulator. As a rule, 4 to 6 lpm is sufficient. The regulator should never be turned above 6 lpm.

Yes: ❑ Reteach: ❑ Return: ❑ Instructor initials: ________

Step 4: The nasal prongs should be gently introduced into the nostrils, so that they appear to be lying on the floor of the nostril.

Yes: ❑ Reteach: ❑ Return: ❑ Instructor initials: ________

Step 5: The tubing should be draped over the ears and cinched loosely under the chin with the ring. The nasal cannula should not be draped over like a necklace; the danger of strangulation is too great. The EMT would then adjust the liter flow to ensure that the patient is receiving an adequate amount.

Yes: ❑ Reteach: ❑ Return: ❑ Instructor initials: ________

Chapter 8 Skill Sheet

Student Name ______________________________ Date ________________

Skill 8-4: Use of a Pocket Mask

Equipment Needed:

1. Pocket mask with oxygen inlet
2. One-way valve
3. Oxygen tubing
4. Oxygen tank
5. Oxygen regulator
6. Gloves
7. Goggles

Yes: ❑ Reteach: ❑ Return: ❑ Instructor initials: ________

Step 1: First, the EMT must ensure that the oxygen tank and oxygen regulator are correctly assembled. The oxygen tank should have sufficient pressure to provide continuous oxygen flow.

Yes: ❑ Reteach: ❑ Return: ❑ Instructor initials: ________

Step 2: Then the EMT chooses the correct oxygen administration device. A pocket mask with an oxygen outlet is preferred when one EMT must ventilate an apneic patient alone.

Yes: ❑ Reteach: ❑ Return: ❑ Instructor initials: ________

Step 3: To use the pocket mask, the EMT must attach the oxygen tubing from the pocket mask to the regulator and turn on the regulator. As a rule, 10 to 15 liters per minute is sufficient.

Yes: ❑ Reteach: ❑ Return: ❑ Instructor initials: ________

Step 4: The EMT then places the apex of the mask over the bridge of the nose and lays the mask over the patient's nose and mouth. An oropharyngeal airway (OPA) should already be in place.

Yes: ❑ Reteach: ❑ Return: ❑ Instructor initials: ________

(continues)

Chapter 8 Skill Sheet

Skill 8-4: *Continued*

Step 5: The EMT then uses a two-handed grasp around the chimney of the mask while grasping the jaw with the remaining fingers.

Yes: ❑ Reteach: ❑ Return: ❑ Instructor initials: ________

Step 6: Tilting the head backward and pulling the jaw upward, the EMT blows into the mask for about 1½ to 2 seconds. The EMT should repeat ventilation every 5 seconds.

Yes: ❑ Reteach: ❑ Return: ❑ Instructor initials: ________

Chapter 8 Skill Sheet

Student Name ______________________________ Date ________________

Skill 8-5: Ventilation with a Bag-Valve-Mask

Equipment Needed:

1. Bag-valve-mask (BVM) assembly
2. Oxygen tubing
3. Oxygen regulator
4. Oxygen tank
5. Gloves
6. Goggles
7. Mask

Yes: ❑ Reteach: ❑ Return: ❑ Instructor initials: ________

Step 1: The EMT must ensure that the oxygen tank and oxygen regulator are correctly assembled. The oxygen tank should have sufficient pressure to provide continuous oxygen flow.

Yes: ❑ Reteach: ❑ Return: ❑ Instructor initials: ________

Step 2: The EMT then chooses the correct oxygen administration device. A BVM assembly is used when an apneic patient needs to be ventilated by two EMTs.

Yes: ❑ Reteach: ❑ Return: ❑ Instructor initials: ________

Step 3: To use the BVM, the EMT must first attach the oxygen tubing to the regulator and turn on the regulator. As a rule, 10 to 15 lpm are sufficient.

Yes: ❑ Reteach: ❑ Return: ❑ Instructor initials: ________

Step 4: The EMT chooses a properly fitting facemask. The facemask should fit securely over the bridge of the nose and extend to the cleft of the chin.

Yes: ❑ Reteach: ❑ Return: ❑ Instructor initials: ________

Step 5: Ensuring that the airway has been opened and an oral airway is in place, the EMT places the mask over the apneic patient's face.

Yes: ❑ Reteach: ❑ Return: ❑ Instructor initials: ________

Step 6: One EMT holds the mask in place using the two-handed "OK" grasp while another EMT compresses the bag with two hands. The patient should be ventilated every 5 seconds.

Yes: ❑ Reteach: ❑ Return: ❑ Instructor initials: ________

Chapter 8 Skill Sheet

Student Name ______________________________ Date ________________

Skill 8-6: Ventilation with a Flow-Restricted Oxygen-Powered Ventilation Device

Equipment Needed:

1. Flow-restricted oxygen-powered ventilation device (FROPVD)
2. Oxygen regulator
3. Oxygen tank
4. Gloves
5. Goggles

Yes: ❑ Reteach: ❑ Return: ❑ Instructor initials: ________

Step 1: The EMT must first ensure that the oxygen tank and oxygen regulator, with the FROPVD, are correctly assembled. The oxygen tank should show sufficient pressure to provide continuous oxygen flow. Then the EMT chooses the correct oxygen administration device. An FROPVD is used when an apneic patient needs to be ventilated by a single EMT.

Yes: ❑ Reteach: ❑ Return: ❑ Instructor initials: ________

Step 2: The EMT should then choose a properly fitting facemask. The facemask should fit securely over the bridge of the nose and extend to the cleft of the chin.

Yes: ❑ Reteach: ❑ Return: ❑ Instructor initials: ________

Step 3: Ensuring that the airway has been opened and an oral airway is in place, the EMT should place the mask over the apneic patient's face.

Yes: ❑ Reteach: ❑ Return: ❑ Instructor initials: ________

Step 4: The patient's head should then be tilted backward.

Yes: ❑ Reteach: ❑ Return: ❑ Instructor initials: ________

Step 5: The EMT holds the mask in place, using the two-handed "OK" grasp while compressing the trigger of the FROPVD for about 2 seconds or until the lungs rise. The patient should be ventilated every 5 seconds.

Yes: ❑ Reteach: ❑ Return: ❑ Instructor initials: ________

(continues)

NREMT Skill Sheet

Oxygen Administration

Start Time: ____________________

Stop Time: ____________________ **Date:** ____________

Candidate's Name: ____________________

Evaluator's Name: ____________________

	Points Possible	Points Awarded
Takes, or verbalizes, body substance isolation precautions	1	
Assembles the regulator to the tank	1	
Opens the tank	1	
Checks for leaks	1	
Checks tank pressure	1	
Attaches non-rebreather mask to oxygen	1	
Prefills reservoir	1	
Adjusts liter flow to 12 liters per minute or greater	1	
Applies and adjusts the mask to the patient's face	1	
Note: The examiner must advise the candidate that the patient is not tolerating the non-rebreather mask. The medical director has ordered you to apply a nasal cannula to the patient.		
Attaches nasal cannula to oxygen	1	
Adjusts liter flow to six (6) liters per minute or less	1	
Applies nasal cannula to the patient	1	
Note: The examiner must advise the candidate to discontinue oxygen therapy.		
Removes the nasal cannula from the patient	1	
Shuts off the regulator	1	
Relieves the pressure within the regulator	1	
Total:	15	

Critical Criteria

_______ Did not take, or verbalize, body substance isolation precautions

_______ Did not assemble the tank and regulator without leaks

_______ Did not prefill the reservoir bag

_______ Did not adjust the device to the correct liter flow for the non-rebreather mask *(12 liters per minute or greater)*

_______ Did not adjust the device to the correct liter flow for the nasal cannula *(6 liters per minute or less)*

NREMT Skill Sheet

Bag-Valve-Mask: Apneic Patient

Start Time: ____________________

Stop Time: ____________________ **Date:** ____________________

Candidate's Name: ____________________

Evaluator's Name: ____________________

	Points Possible	Points Awarded
Takes, or verbalizes, body substance isolation precautions	1	
Voices opening the airway	1	
Voices inserting an airway adjunct	1	
Selects appropriately sized mask	1	
Creates a proper mask-to-face seal	1	
Ventilates patient at no less than 800 ml volume ***(The examiner must witness for at least 30 seconds)***	1	
Connects reservoir and oxygen	1	
Adjusts liter flow to 15 liters/minute or greater	1	
The examiner indicates arrival of a second EMT. The second EMT is instructed to ventilate the patient while the candidate controls the mask and the airway		
Voices re-opening the airway	1	
Creates a proper mask-to-face seal	1	
Instructs assistant to resume ventilation at proper volume per breath ***(The examiner must witness for at least 30 seconds)***	1	
Total:	11	

Critical Criteria

_______ Did not take, or verbalize, body substance isolation precautions

_______ Did not immediately ventilate the patient

_______ Interrupted ventilations for more than 20 seconds

_______ Did not provide high concentration of oxygen

_______ Did not provide, or direct assistant to provide, proper volume/breath
(more than two (2) ventilations per minute are below 800 ml)

_______ Did not allow adequate exhalation

CHAPTER 9
Shock: A State of Hypoperfusion

Cells in the body require oxygen to function properly. When they are without oxygen for a period of time, they are not able to function and will eventually die. The EMT-B must be able to recognize compensated shock and set management priorities.

Missing Letters: Complete the puzzle using the Key Terms in Chapter 9 of the textbook.

h _ _ _ _ _ _ _ _ _ _   _ _ _ _ _

_ y _ _ _ _ _ _ _ _

p _ _ _

_ _ _ o _ _   _ _ _ _ _ _

_ _ _ _ _ p _ _ _ _ _ _ _

e _ _ _ _ _ _ _ _ _ _ _

_ _ _ _ _ _ r _ _ _ _ _   _ _ _ _ _

_ _ _ f _ _ _ _ _

u _ _ _ _ _ _ _ _

_ _ _ _ _ _ s _ _ _ _

_ _ _ _ i _ _ _ _ _ _   _ _ _ _ _

_ _ _ _ _ _ _ o _ _ _ _ _

_ _ _ _ _ _ _ n _ _   _ _ _ _ _

Identification: Read the following and determine the type of shock in each case. Write the type on the line in front of the case.

1. ______________ A patient bleeds profusely.
2. ______________ A child has excessive nausea, vomiting, and diarrhea.
3. ______________ A diabetic patient has an excessive amount of urination.
4. ______________ A runner sweats profusely.
5. ______________ A child, allergic to nuts, eats peanut brittle.
6. ______________ A patient has a bacterial infection.
7. ______________ A patient is stung by a wasp.
8. ______________ A patient falls from a ladder onto his back.
9. ______________ A patient develops a severe heart attack.

Ordering: Place in order from the first organ to lose perfusion to the last. Place a numeral 1 before the first, 2 before the next, and so on.

_____ brain

_____ abdominal organs

_____ skin, muscles, bones, and uterus

_____ heart and lungs

Identification: Read each set of signs and symptoms for an adult patient and decide if the set describes compensated or decompensated shock. Write the correct answer on the line in front of each.

1. ______________________ Pale, respiratory rate elevated, BP normal
2. ______________________ Cold, gray, unconscious, can't hear BP
3. ______________________ Confused, rapid pulse, BP low
4. ______________________ Anxious, BP normal, very fast pulse
5. ______________________ Thirsty, strong pulses at the wrist
6. ______________________ Nauseous, fast respirations, BP normal
7. ______________________ Agitated, BP normal, cool, pale
8. ______________________ No pulses at wrist, can't hear BP, cool

True or False: Read each statement and decide if it is true or false. Place T or F on the line before each statement.

1. _____ Perfusion describes bringing oxygen into the lungs.
2. _____ Hypoperfusion means delivery of oxygenated blood to tissues is less than is necessary or not occurring.
3. _____ Lymph is the fluid part of the cardiovascular system.
4. _____ Capillaries can alter their diameter by contraction or relaxation of muscles.
5. _____ Increased respiratory rate is one of the body's compensatory mechanisms.
6. _____ Once the systolic BP drops to less than 90 mm Hg, irreversible shock results.
7. _____ As perfusion to the skin decreases, capillary refill time will increase.
8. _____ It is not necessary to reassess a patient's mental status beyond that done initially.
9. _____ A drop in blood pressure associated with a change in position is called a positive tilt test.
10. _____ Use of the MAST/PASG is contraindicated in pelvic fractures.

Short Answer: Read each question. Think about the information presented in your text, and then answer each question with one or two sentences.

1. Which type(s) of shock are caused by the inability of the blood vessels to constrict?

2. Which type(s) of shock are due to fluid loss?

3. Which type(s) of shock are caused by the inability of the heart to pump?

4. Should MAST/PASG be removed by the EMT-B? Why or why not?

5. How often should a patient experiencing hypoperfusion be monitored?

Critical Thinking 1: Read each scenario and then answer the questions.

Cindy and Paul arrived at the Reams home for the 6-month-old daughter who has a "stomach bug" according to her mother. The child, Brittany, had been vomiting and having diarrhea for two days. Her mother had been trying to get her to drink small amounts of liquids but called EMS when she noticed that there were no wet diapers. Cindy performed an initial assessment while Paul gathered a history.

1. What important observations must Cindy make at this time?

2. Why is the child's response to her mother an important observation?

3. Explain the normal blood pressure result.

4. How should Cindy and Paul proceed?

Critical Thinking 2: Read each scenario and then answer the questions.

Mrs. Evers called EMS because she had been very weak and dizzy. She was afraid that she would fall and injure herself. When Julie and Serge arrived, they found Mrs. Evers lying pale, cool, and clammy, on her couch. Julie obtained a history while Serge performed an initial assessment and began treatment. Mrs. Evers had a history of arthritis. Her doctor had started her on a new medicine that could cause bleeding in the stomach. Julie discovered that Mrs. Evers had been vomiting some material that looked like old blood and that her stools (bowel movements) had been very dark.

1. In addition to the usual baseline vital signs, what added assessment might Julie and Serge want to obtain?

2. How should Julie and Serge treat Mrs. Evers?

Critical Thinking 3: Read each scenario and then answer the questions.

Brenda and Jerry responded to an incident where a man had fallen from a porch roof approximately 6 feet off the ground. When they arrived, the man was lying on his back on the ground. He was flushed and had a number of raised reddened areas on his trunk and arms. He also was breathing fast, and a high pitched whistle was noted with each breath. A pulse could not be found at the wrist.

1. What is the likely cause of the inability to find a pulse at the wrists?

2. What are the raised reddened areas called?

3. What treatments should Brenda and Jerry provide?

Chapter 9 Skill Sheet

Student Name ______________________________ Date ______________

Skill 9-1: Orthostatic Vital Signs

Equipment Needed:

1. Stethoscope
2. Blood pressure cuff
3. Watch with second hand
4. Gloves

Yes: ❑ Reteach: ❑ Return: ❑ Instructor initials: ________

Step 1: Obtain a full set of vital signs from the supine patient.

Yes: ❑ Reteach: ❑ Return: ❑ Instructor initials: ________

Step 2: Assist the patient to standing, with an assistant behind the patient.

Yes: ❑ Reteach: ❑ Return: ❑ Instructor initials: ________

Step 3: Repeat vital signs.

Yes: ❑ Reteach: ❑ Return: ❑ Instructor initials: ________

Step 4: Compare vital signs lying and standing.

Yes: ❑ Reteach: ❑ Return: ❑ Instructor initials: ________

Step 5: Treat for shock as indicated. Record or report significant changes.

Yes: ❑ Reteach: ❑ Return: ❑ Instructor initials: ________

Chapter 9 Skill Sheet

Student Name ______________________________ Date ________________

Skill 9-2: Application of MAST/PASG

Equipment Needed:

1. MAST/PASG with foot pump attachment
2. Stethoscope
3. Blood pressure cuff
4. Patient Care Report and pen
5. Gloves

Yes: ❑ Reteach: ❑ Return: ❑ Instructor initials: ________

Step 1: Perform initial assessment and vital signs. Identify indications for MAST/PASG application: injured patient with severe hypotension (SBP < 50 mm Hg) or hypotension (SBP < 90 mm Hg) with associated pelvic instability with other signs of shock (>2 of the following: altered mental status, persistent tachycardia, cool and clammy skin, diaphoresis, thirst, or nausea).

Yes: ❑ Reteach: ❑ Return: ❑ Instructor initials: ________

Step 2: Ensure lack of absolute contraindications (pulmonary edema or penetrating chest injury) and relative contraindications (pregnancy, impaled object, evisceration).

Yes: ❑ Reteach: ❑ Return: ❑ Instructor initials: ________

Step 3: Pull MAST/PASG up to the level of the lower ribs and secure Velcro fasteners.

Yes: ❑ Reteach: ❑ Return: ❑ Instructor initials: ________

Step 4: Attach air hoses and set to open position. Use foot pump to inflate trousers until gauge reaches 106 mm Hg or pop-off valve releases. All valves should be opened and in-line.

Yes: ❑ Reteach: ❑ Return: ❑ Instructor initials: ________

Step 5: Set air pump hoses to closed position. Reassess patient's ABCs and vital signs.

Yes: ❑ Reteach: ❑ Return: ❑ Instructor initials: ________

(continues)

NREMT Skill Sheet

Bleeding Control/Shock Management

Start Time: ______________________________

Stop Time: ______________________________ **Date:** ____________________

Candidate's Name: ____

Evaluator's Name: ____

	Points Possible	Points Awarded
Takes, or verbalizes, body substance isolation precautions	1	
Applies direct pressure to the wound	1	
Evaluates the extremity	1	
Note: The examiner must now inform the candidate that the wound continues to bleed.		
Applies an additional dressing to the wound	1	
Note: The examiner must now inform the candidate that the wound still continues to bleed. The second dressing does not control the bleeding.		
Locates and applies pressure to appropriate arterial pressure point	1	
Note: The examiner must now inform the candidate that the bleeding is controlled.		
Bandages the wound	1	
Note: The examiner must now inform the candidate the patient is now showing signs and symptoms indicative of hypoperfusion.		
Properly positions the patient	1	
Applies high concentration oxygen	1	
Initiates steps to prevent heat loss from the patient	1	
Indicates the need for immediate transportation	1	
Total:	10	

Critical Criteria

_______ Did not take, or verbalize, body substance isolation precautions

_______ Did not apply high concentration of oxygen

_______ Applied a tourniquet before attempting other methods of bleeding control

_______ Did not control hemorrhage in a timely manner

_______ Did not indicate a need for immediate transportation

CHAPTER 10 Baseline Vital Signs and SAMPLE History

During the course of training, the EMT-B will learn many skills. The skills used most frequently are obtaining vital signs and gathering a basic patient history.

Definitions: Define the following terms.

1. anisocoria ______________________________
2. cyanosis ______________________________
3. constricted ______________________________
4. jaundice ______________________________
5. dilated ______________________________
6. pallor ______________________________
7. diastolic ______________________________
8. PERRL ______________________________
9. systolic ______________________________
10. sphygmomanometer ______________________________

Matching: Match each word or term with its definition.

1. _____	inspiration	a.	nostrils opening widely with each breath
2. _____	exhalation	b.	harsh inspiratory sound
3. _____	pulse oximeter	c.	noise caused by blockage with the tongue
4. _____	stridor	d.	neck and chest muscles
5. _____	gurgling	e.	breathing in
6. _____	snoring	f.	high-pitched inspiratory or expiratory sound
7. _____	wheezing	g.	device to measure oxygen on the RBCs
8. _____	grunting	h.	breathing out
9. _____	accessory muscles	i.	noise from liquid in the airway
10. _____	nasal flaring	j.	noise from extreme effort to breathe

Calculation: Calculate the following respiratory rates.

1. 15 breaths in 30 seconds = ________ breaths per minute
2. 10 breaths in 30 seconds = ________ breaths per minute
3. 24 breaths in 60 seconds = ________ breaths per minute
4. 6 breaths in 30 seconds = ________ breaths per minute

Calculation: Calculate the following pulse rates.

1. 32 beats in 30 seconds = __________ beats per minute
2. 45 beats in 30 seconds = __________ beats per minute

3. 68 beats in 60 seconds = __________ beats per minute
4. 90 beats in 60 seconds = __________ beats per minute
5. 52 beats in 30 seconds = __________ beats per minute

True or False: Read each statement and decide if it is true or false. Place T or F on the line before each statement.

1. _____ The systolic pressure measures the heart at rest.
2. _____ Diastolic pressure measures force in the arteries during cardiac relaxation.
3. _____ A cuff that covers one-third of the upper arm is the correct size.
4. _____ To auscultate a blood pressure, the EMT-B will need a stethoscope.
5. _____ Palpating a blood pressure is more accurate than auscultation.

Sorting: Complete the following table of skin signs by placing the descriptor in the correct column.

cool | pallor
jaundice | hot
sweaty | cyanosis
flushed | gray
pink | warm
dry

Color	Temperature	Condition

Identification: Read each of the following and determine if it describes a sign or a symptom. Place the correct word on the line in front of the term.

1. ______________ Pulse of 92 beats per minute
2. ______________ "I can't breathe"
3. ______________ Leg pain
4. ______________ Tenderness when touched
5. ______________ Accessory muscle use
6. ______________ Grunting respirations
7. ______________ Nausea
8. ______________ Vomiting
9. ______________ Cyanosis
10. ______________ 22 breaths per minute
11. ______________ Dizzy
12. ______________ Chest pain

13. ________________ Dry skin
14. ________________ Sweaty
15. ________________ Headache

Sorting: Read the following patient story. Place the information into the correct SAMPLE category.

Mr. Jones called EMS because he was having difficulty breathing. He sat in the tripod position and used accessory muscles to breathe. Normally, his inhaler of Ventolin helped but today it didn't. He wanted his doctor to order more medications but at present only had the inhaler. He was taking vitamins and a daily aspirin to help him feel better. His doctor had told him that he had lung disease caused by many years of smoking. Also, eggs caused him to break out in hives. He used his inhaler one hour before calling EMS and had eaten breakfast that morning. The hot and humid weather always seemed to bother him.

S

A

M

P

L

E

Chapter 10 Skill Sheet

Student Name ________________________________ Date ________________

Skill 10-1: Measurement of Respiration

Equipment Needed:

1. Watch/clock with second hand
2. Patient Care Report and pen
3. Gloves

Yes: ❑ Reteach: ❑ Return: ❑ Instructor initials: ________

Step 1: The EMT places her hand on top of the patient's hand, then places the patient's hand on top of the abdomen. Apply any appropriate personal protective equipment. Observe patient's chest or abdomen for rise and fall with respiration, noting any irregular patterns, noises, or effort. Note whether the respiration is shallow or particularly labored.

Yes: ❑ Reteach: ❑ Return: ❑ Instructor initials: ________

Step 2: Count the number of complete breaths taken (one inspiration and one exhalation counts as *one* breath) over a 30-second period.

Yes: ❑ Reteach: ❑ Return: ❑ Instructor initials: ________

Step 3: Multiply this number by 2 to obtain breaths per minute.

Yes: ❑ Reteach: ❑ Return: ❑ Instructor initials: ________

Step 4: The EMT should consider taking a pulse oximetry reading at this time.

Yes: ❑ Reteach: ❑ Return: ❑ Instructor initials: ________

Step 5: Record the respiratory rate and quality.

Yes: ❑ Reteach: ❑ Return: ❑ Instructor initials: ________

Chapter 10 Skill Sheet

Student Name ______________________________ Date ________________

Skill 10-2: Measurement of Radial Pulse

Equipment Needed:

1. Watch/clock with second hand
2. Patient Care Report and pen
3. Gloves

Yes: ❑ Reteach: ❑ Return: ❑ Instructor initials: ________

Step 1: First, the EMT notes the condition of the skin as warm or cool, and moist or dry.

Yes: ❑ Reteach: ❑ Return: ❑ Instructor initials: ________

Step 2: Next, the EMT finds the radial pulse. The radial pulse is on the anterior surface of the distal forearm, proximal to the thumb. The EMT notes the quality and regularity of the pulse as weak or strong, regular or irregular.

Yes: ❑ Reteach: ❑ Return: ❑ Instructor initials: ________

Step 3: The EMT then counts the number of pulse beats felt over a 30-second period. (If the pulse is irregular, then the EMT counts for 1 minute.)

Yes: ❑ Reteach: ❑ Return: ❑ Instructor initials: ________

Step 4: Multiply this number by 2 to obtain beats per minute.

Yes: ❑ Reteach: ❑ Return: ❑ Instructor initials: ________

Step 5: Record quality and regularity of the pulse rate and the condition of the skin.

Yes: ❑ Reteach: ❑ Return: ❑ Instructor initials: ________

Chapter 10 Skill Sheet

Student Name ______________________________ Date ________________

Skill 10-3: Measurement of Blood Pressure by Auscultation

Equipment Needed:

1. Stethoscope
2. Properly sized blood pressure cuff
3. Gloves

Yes: ❑ Reteach: ❑ Return: ❑ Instructor initials: ________

Step 1: The EMT places the blood pressure cuff snugly around the patient's upper arm. The cuff should cover more than half but less than two-thirds of the length of the upper arm.

Yes: ❑ Reteach: ❑ Return: ❑ Instructor initials: ________

Step 2: The EMT then finds the brachial pulse. The brachial pulse is usually found on the medial side of the elbow.

Yes: ❑ Reteach: ❑ Return: ❑ Instructor initials: ________

Step 3: Next, the EMT closes the valve on the cuff and inflates the cuff until the brachial pulse is no longer felt, then continues inflating for 20 mm Hg higher.

Yes: ❑ Reteach: ❑ Return: ❑ Instructor initials: ________

Step 4: Then the EMT places the head of the stethoscope on the brachial pulse and the ear tips in the ears.

Yes: ❑ Reteach: ❑ Return: ❑ Instructor initials: ________

Step 5: Slowly deflate the blood pressure cuff, at about 10 mm Hg per second, using the valve next to the bulb.

Yes: ❑ Reteach: ❑ Return: ❑ Instructor initials: ________

Step 6: Note the systolic and the diastolic pressures.

Yes: ❑ Reteach: ❑ Return: ❑ Instructor initials: ________

Chapter 10 Skill Sheet

Student Name ________________________________ Date _______________

Skill 10-4: Measurement of Blood Pressure by Palpation

Equipment Needed:

1. Properly sized blood pressure cuff
2. Gloves

Yes: ❑ Reteach: ❑ Return: ❑ Instructor initials: ________

Step 1: The EMT places the blood pressure cuff snugly around the patient's upper arm. The cuff should cover more than half but less than two-thirds of the length of the upper arm.

Yes: ❑ Reteach: ❑ Return: ❑ Instructor initials: ________

Step 2: The EMT then finds the brachial pulse. The brachial pulse is usually found on the medial side of the elbow.

Yes: ❑ Reteach: ❑ Return: ❑ Instructor initials: ________

Step 3: Next, the EMT closes the valve on the cuff and inflates the cuff until the brachial pulse is no longer felt, then continues inflating for 20 mm Hg higher.

Yes: ❑ Reteach: ❑ Return: ❑ Instructor initials: ________

Step 4: Then the EMT places her fingertips over the radial pulse and slowly deflates the blood pressure cuff until the pulse returns.

Yes: ❑ Reteach: ❑ Return: ❑ Instructor initials: ________

Step 5: The EMT notes the pressure on the valve at the time that she felt the return of the radial pulse.

Yes: ❑ Reteach: ❑ Return: ❑ Instructor initials: ________

Step 6: The EMT records the reading on the Patient Care Report.

Yes: ❑ Reteach: ❑ Return: ❑ Instructor initials: ________

Chapter 10 Skill Sheet

Student Name ______________________________ Date ________________

Skill 10-5: Pulse Oximetry

Equipment Needed:

1. Pulse oximeter with indicator light
2. Nail polish remover
3. Gloves

Yes: ❑ Reteach: ❑ Return: ❑ Instructor initials: ________

Step 1: Assess the patient. Never withhold oxygen to obtain an oxygen saturation if the patient is hypoxic.

Yes: ❑ Reteach: ❑ Return: ❑ Instructor initials: ________

Step 2: Turn on the pulse oximeter and check for self-test results.

Yes: ❑ Reteach: ❑ Return: ❑ Instructor initials: ________

Step 3: Place the probe on patient's finger (if nail polish is present, remove the polish first).

Yes: ❑ Reteach: ❑ Return: ❑ Instructor initials: ________

Step 4: If distal circulation is diminished, place a disposable probe over the bridge of the nose.

Yes: ❑ Reteach: ❑ Return: ❑ Instructor initials: ________

Step 5: Check the indicator light, ensuring adequate sampling. Note the reading as "percent saturated" and document it.

Yes: ❑ Reteach: ❑ Return: ❑ Instructor initials: ________

CHAPTER 11
Lifting and Moving Patients

Packaging, lifting, and carrying occurs on every EMS call. It is one of the fundamental aspects of EMS that has not changed over time.

Definitions: The following are methods for lifting and moving patients. Choose the correct one from the list and place it on the line.

arm drag	end-to-end stretcher carry
blanket drag	extremity carry
caterpillar pass	firefighter's carry
clothing drag	firefighter's drag
cradle carry	pack strap carry
diamond stretcher carry	power lift
direct carry	rescuer assist
direct lift	seat carry
emergency moves	squat lift

1. ________________ A carry in which the patient's arms are around the EMT's neck and the EMT crawls with the patient's body underneath
2. ________________ A technique used by a single EMT to help a patient to walk
3. ________________ A method of movement in which the EMT-B grasps the patient's wrists and pulls the arms back over the patient's head
4. ________________ A carry in which the EMT-B grasps the patient's arms and hoists the patient onto his back with the feet dragging
5. ________________ A method of carrying a stretcher in which there is an EMT-B on each end plus one on each side
6. ________________ A carry in which two EMT-Bs lock arms and allow the patient to sit on their arms
7. ________________ Two EMT-Bs, one on each end of the stretcher, carry it
8. ________________ A means to replace tired EMT-Bs with rested ones without lowering the stretcher
9. ________________ Also called a power lift
10. ________________ Technique that involves lifting a patient up onto the EMT-B's shoulders to quickly move her from a dangerous environment
11. ________________ A technique used to lift a heavy object from the ground
12. ________________ Use of collar or handful of clothing to quickly remove a patient from a dangerous scene
13. ________________ A technique that allows three EMT-Bs to lift a patient from the ground without using assistive devices
14. ________________ Methods that allow an EMT-B to rapidly remove a patient in an emergency
15. ________________ Lifting a person and carrying her a short distance to a stretcher
16. ________________ Placing a patient on a blanket and dragging it over the ground

17. ________________ Holding a patient in one's arms and carrying her for a rapid move
18. ________________ Two EMT-Bs lift the patient under arms and knees

Matching: Match each word or term with its definition.

1. _____	flexible stretcher	a.	protection over rough terrain
2. _____	cravat	b.	sturdy linen for transferring a patient
3. _____	draw sheet	c.	plastic stretcher that rolls up when unused
4. _____	stairchair	d.	commercial flexible stretcher
5. _____	transfer board	e.	can be separated for placement
6. _____	basket stretcher	f.	also called a slide board
7. _____	Reeves stretcher	g.	triangular cotton dressing
8. _____	scoop stretcher	h.	with wheels for moving a seated patient

Identification: Read each scenario and decide which require an emergency move. Place a checkmark on the line before those that require an emergency move.

1. _______ Person stuck in a car; complaining of leg pain
2. _______ Person unconscious from smoke in a fireworks factory
3. _______ Person with a fractured leg is lying across a patient in respiratory arrest
4. _______ The driver of a car smashed her face and knocked out several teeth; airway patent
5. _______ Person is still inside a vehicle that has overturned into a creek
6. _______ A person is complaining of back and leg pain
7. _______ A person has bleeding from a head laceration
8. _______ A person is complaining of mild shortness of breath following a fender bender
9. _______ A person collapses outside a building where there is a gas leak
10. _______ A person is in respiratory arrest following a minor accident

Short Answer: Read each question. Think about the information presented in your text, and then answer each question with one or two sentences.

1. What region of the spine is likely to suffer an injury from improper lifting or moving?

2. Why do exercises help prevent back injury?

3. The EMT-B needs to lift the extrication tools from the floor. The tools weigh 45 pounds. Describe the correct way to lift them.

4. A patient must be moved onto a hospital stretcher. Describe two ways in which an EMT-B can accomplish this safely.

5. Deanna is afraid she will injure her back, so she has chosen to wear a back support tightly whenever she is on duty. Explain how this choice could actually cause Deanna to have an injury.

Critical Thinking: Read each scenario and then decide how to move the patient from scene to ambulance.

1. George, Jason, and Steve were called to the Johnson residence for Mrs. Johnson, who had fallen. Mrs. Johnson was a fiercely independent woman who took pride in running her small Mom and Pop grocery store, even at age 78. Upon their arrival, they found Mrs. Johnson lying on her right side in a cramped narrow aisle. She stated that she was turning around quickly, felt a "snap" at her hip, and couldn't stay standing. She lowered herself to the floor but now couldn't move due to the pain in her right leg and hip.

2. Corinne, Rebekah, and Tim answered a cell phone call for a "man down" at the local high school. Once there, they found Mr. Joli, the janitor. He said that he had been readying cleaners to really clean the area before graduation and had tripped over a bucket, falling forward onto his arms. His arms hurt, and his right leg was deformed and very painful. Worse, the chemicals had spilled and were very slowly running toward one another.

3. Ted and Katie are called to the third-floor walk-up of Mrs. Hedderman. They find her seated upright in a chair, having trouble breathing.

Chapter 11 Skill Sheet

Student Name ______________________________ Date ______________

Skill 11-1: Proper Lifting Techniques

Equipment Needed:

1. Appropriate PPE
2. Appropriate back support
3. Proper footwear
4. Adequate numbers of trained assistants

Yes: ❑ Reteach: ❑ Return: ❑ Instructor initials: ________

Step 1: The EMT positions his feet about shoulder length apart, facing forward.

Yes: ❑ Reteach: ❑ Return: ❑ Instructor initials: ________

Step 2: The EMT then lowers his body by bending at knees, one knee down, keeping back straight.

Yes: ❑ Reteach: ❑ Return: ❑ Instructor initials: ________

Step 3: Grasping the object with both hands, palms upward (power grip), the EMT lifts evenly and smoothly.

Yes: ❑ Reteach: ❑ Return: ❑ Instructor initials: ________

Step 4: With arms locked out straight, the EMT stands fully upright.

Yes: ❑ Reteach: ❑ Return: ❑ Instructor initials: ________

Chapter 11 Skill Sheet

Student Name ______________________________ Date ________________

Skill 11-2: The Clothing Drag

Equipment Needed:

Appropriate PPE

Yes: ❑ Reteach: ❑ Return: ❑ Instructor initials: ________

Step 1: The EMT grasps the patient's clothing at the collar, while cradling the patient's head on his forearms.

Yes: ❑ Reteach: ❑ Return: ❑ Instructor initials: ________

Step 2: Crouching down, with back straight, the EMT walks backward.

Yes: ❑ Reteach: ❑ Return: ❑ Instructor initials: ________

Chapter 11 Skill Sheet

Student Name ______________________________ Date ________________

Skill 11-3: The Arm Drag

Equipment Needed:

Appropriate PPE

Yes: ❑ Reteach: ❑ Return: ❑ Instructor initials: ________

Step 1: Kneeling down, the EMT slides his arms under the patient's arms and grasps the wrists across the chest.

Yes: ❑ Reteach: ❑ Return: ❑ Instructor initials: ________

Step 2: Standing up, the EMT walks backward.

Yes: ❑ Reteach: ❑ Return: ❑ Instructor initials: ________

Chapter 11 Skill Sheet

Student Name ______________________________ Date ________________

Skill 11-4: The Blanket Drag

Equipment Needed:

1. Appropriate PPE
2. Blanket, tarp, drape, or similar covering

Yes: ❑ Reteach: ❑ Return: ❑ Instructor initials: ________

Step 1: Place the blanket along the long axis of the body, leaving about one foot of material at the head.

Yes: ❑ Reteach: ❑ Return: ❑ Instructor initials: ________

Step 2: Logroll the patient onto the blanket, pulling the blanket from underneath the patient.

Yes: ❑ Reteach: ❑ Return: ❑ Instructor initials: ________

Step 3: Wrap the patient with the blanket, protecting the patient.

Yes: ❑ Reteach: ❑ Return: ❑ Instructor initials: ________

Step 4: Roll up the excess material at the head and grasp the roll.

Yes: ❑ Reteach: ❑ Return: ❑ Instructor initials: ________

Chapter 11 Skill Sheet

Student Name ______________________________ Date ________________

Skill 11-5: The Firefighter's Drag

Equipment Needed:

1. Appropriate PPE
2. Triangular bandage

Yes: ❑ Reteach: ❑ Return: ❑ Instructor initials: ________

Step 1: Using the triangular bandage, folded into a cravat, the EMT secures the patient's wrists together.

Yes: ❑ Reteach: ❑ Return: ❑ Instructor initials: ________

Step 2: While on all fours, the EMT drapes the tied hands over his shoulders and drags the patient underneath him.

Yes: ❑ Reteach: ❑ Return: ❑ Instructor initials: ________

Chapter 11 Skill Sheet

Student Name ____________________ Date ____________

Skill 11-6: The Rescuer Assist

Equipment Needed:

Appropriate PPE

Yes: ❑ Reteach: ❑ Return: ❑ Instructor initials: ________

Step 1: The EMT crouches to the patient's level and swings one arm over the EMT's shoulders.

Yes: ❑ Reteach: ❑ Return: ❑ Instructor initials: ________

Step 2: With one hand grasping the patient's beltline, and another grasping the patient's other wrist, the EMT stands and assists the patient with walking.

Yes: ❑ Reteach: ❑ Return: ❑ Instructor initials: ________

Chapter 11 Skill Sheet

Student Name ______________________________ Date ________________

Skill 11-7: The Pack Strap Carry

Equipment Needed:

Appropriate PPE

Yes: ❑ Reteach: ❑ Return: ❑ Instructor initials: ________

Step 1: Crouching in front of the seated patient, grasp the patient's wrists and pivot on the heels, draping the patient's arms over the sholders.

Yes: ❑ Reteach: ❑ Return: ❑ Instructor initials: ________

Step 2: Stand and hoist the patient onto the shoulders and off her feet. (This carry is also useful if the patient who is being assisted suddenly tires and needs to be carried. The EMT would simply release the belt and step in front of the patient, grasping the free hand and placing it over his shoulders.)

Yes: ❑ Reteach: ❑ Return: ❑ Instructor initials: ________

Chapter 11 Skill Sheet

Student Name ______________________ Date ____________

Skill 11-8: The Cradle Carry

Equipment Needed:

Appropriate PPE

Yes: ❑ Reteach: ❑ Return: ❑ Instructor initials: ______

Step 1: The EMT first kneels next to the supine patient, placing one hand under the shoulders and the other hand under the knees.

Yes: ❑ Reteach: ❑ Return: ❑ Instructor initials: ______

Step 2: The EMT then stands, keeping the patient's body close to his.

Yes: ❑ Reteach: ❑ Return: ❑ Instructor initials: ______

Chapter 11 Skill Sheet

Student Name ______________________________ Date ________________

Skill 11-9: The Firefighter's Carry

Equipment Needed:

Appropriate PPE

Yes: ❑ Reteach: ❑ Return: ❑ Instructor initials: ________

Step 1: The EMT starts by standing toe to toe with the supine patient. Crouching down, he grabs the patient's wrists and proceeds to roll the patient to a seated position.

Yes: ❑ Reteach: ❑ Return: ❑ Instructor initials: ________

Step 2: Without stopping, the EMT then pulls the patient as nearly erect as possible.

Yes: ❑ Reteach: ❑ Return: ❑ Instructor initials: ________

Step 3: Quickly crouching again, the EMT places his shoulder into the patient's abdomen, while simultaneously standing.

Yes: ❑ Reteach: ❑ Return: ❑ Instructor initials: ________

Step 4: The EMT then puts one arm through the patient's legs and grasps the patient's hand lying across his chest, effectively locking the patient over his shoulders. (Another EMT may help hoist the patient up onto the shouders of the EMT. The second EMT waits until the patient is up and over the first EMT's shoulders, then, grasping the patient's knee, helps hoist the patient.)

Yes: ❑ Reteach: ❑ Return: ❑ Instructor initials: ________

Chapter 11 Skill Sheet

Student Name ______________________ Date __________

Skill 11-10: The Seat Carry

Equipment Needed:

Appropriate PPE

Yes: ❑ Reteach: ❑ Return: ❑ Instructor initials: ______

Step 1: The two EMTs kneel on opposite knees, and clasp arms. Each EMT should grasp the other EMT at the elbow.

Yes: ❑ Reteach: ❑ Return: ❑ Instructor initials: ______

Step 2: With one pair of arms high, the patient sits back into the seat that has been created. The EMTs then stand together, at the same time.

Yes: ❑ Reteach: ❑ Return: ❑ Instructor initials: ______

Chapter 11 Skill Sheet

Student Name ______________________ Date ____________

Skill 11-11: The Chair Carry

Equipment Needed:

1. Appropriate PPE
2. Hardback chair

Yes: ❑ Reteach: ❑ Return: ❑ Instructor initials: ________

Step 1: The patient is assisted to sitting in the chair.

Yes: ❑ Reteach: ❑ Return: ❑ Instructor initials: ________

Step 2: One EMT kneels in front of the chair, facing forward, and between the patient's legs. He reaches back and grasps the legs of the chair.

Yes: ❑ Reteach: ❑ Return: ❑ Instructor initials: ________

Step 3: The second EMT, at the back of the chair, grasps the uprights of the chair and leans the chair backward.

Yes: ❑ Reteach: ❑ Return: ❑ Instructor initials: ________

Step 4: Simultaneously, the two EMTs lift the patient up and proceed to walk forward together.

Yes: ❑ Reteach: ❑ Return: ❑ Instructor initials: ________

Chapter 11 Skill Sheet

Student Name ______________________ Date ____________

Skill 11-12: The Extremity Lift

Equipment Needed:

Appropriate PPE

Yes: ❑ Reteach: ❑ Return: ❑ Instructor initials: ________

Step 1: The first EMT kneels behind the patient and helps the patient up to a sitting position. The patient can be rested against the EMTs knee for a moment.

Yes: ❑ Reteach: ❑ Return: ❑ Instructor initials: ________

Step 2: The EMT then reaches under the patient's arms and grasps the patient's wrists, pulling them against the patient's chest tightly.

Yes: ❑ Reteach: ❑ Return: ❑ Instructor initials: ________

Step 3: The second EMT then crouches. Reaching down on each side, the EMT grasps under the patient's knees. (In some cases it may be more convenient to crouch beside the patient's knees and hook arms under the patient's knees.)

Yes: ❑ Reteach: ❑ Return: ❑ Instructor initials: ________

Step 4: Simultaneously, the two EMTs stand with the patient and walk forward together.

Yes: ❑ Reteach: ❑ Return: ❑ Instructor initials: ________

Chapter 11 Skill Sheet

Student Name ______________________________ Date ________________

Skill 11-13: The Direct Lift

Equipment Needed:

Appropriate PPE

Yes: ❑ Reteach: ❑ Return: ❑ Instructor initials: ________

Step 1: Both of the EMTs stand on one side of the supine patient and then kneel, on the same knee, beside the patient.

Yes: ❑ Reteach: ❑ Return: ❑ Instructor initials: ________

Step 2: The first EMT places one arm under the patient's head and neck and the other arm under the shoulders. The second EMT places his arms under the patient's lower back and buttocks.

Yes: ❑ Reteach: ❑ Return: ❑ Instructor initials: ________

Step 3: Simultaneously, the two EMTs hoist the patient to their knees. If the patient is being transferred to a stretcher on the other side of the patient, they need only drop the one knee to move forward and over the stretcher. If the patient is to be carried any distance, the EMTs should roll the patient against their chests and then walk forward together.

Yes: ❑ Reteach: ❑ Return: ❑ Instructor initials: ________

Chapter 11 Skill Sheet

Student Name ____________________ Date ____________

Skill 11-14: The Scoop Stretcher

Equipment Needed:

1. Appropriate PPE
2. Orthopedic stretcher

Yes: ❑ Reteach: ❑ Return: ❑ Instructor initials: ________

Step 1: The scoop stretcher must be split into its two halves, which must be adjusted to the patient's length.

Yes: ❑ Reteach: ❑ Return: ❑ Instructor initials: ________

Step 2: The patient is then logrolled to one side and the scoop stretcher half placed along the patient's axis. This is repeated with the other side, and the two ends are secured.

Yes: ❑ Reteach: ❑ Return: ❑ Instructor initials: ________

Chapter 11 Skill Sheet

Student Name ______________________________ Date ________________

Skill 11-15: Use of a Stringer

Equipment Needed:

1. Appropriate PPE
2. Loop of webbing approximately 6 feet long

Yes: ❑ Reteach: ❑ Return: ❑ Instructor initials: ________

Step 1: The EMT places the webbing under the bar, or handhold, and loops it back through itself, in effect creating a half-hitch.

Yes: ❑ Reteach: ❑ Return: ❑ Instructor initials: ________

Step 2: The EMT then kneels next to the stretcher and slips the loop of webbing over his shoulder, being sure that the webbing knot is not on the shoulder.

Yes: ❑ Reteach: ❑ Return: ❑ Instructor initials: ________

Step 3: Then the EMT slips his opposite hand inside the loop. It may be necessary to shorten the length of the loop by tying a knot in the webbing.

Yes: ❑ Reteach: ❑ Return: ❑ Instructor initials: ________

Step 4: Once standing, the EMT adjusts the loop over his shoulders. One hand should be carrying the stretcher and the other hand should be exerting downward force on the loop, in effect balancing the load.

Yes: ❑ Reteach: ❑ Return: ❑ Instructor initials: ________

Chapter 11 Skill Sheet

Student Name ______________________________ Date ________________

Skill 11-16: The Caterpillar Pass

Equipment Needed:

1. Appropriate PPE
2. Stretcher or litter

Yes: ❑ Reteach: ❑ Return: ❑ Instructor initials: ________

Step 1: Coming to the obstacle, all EMTs stop and turn toward each other. Two EMTs go around or over the obstacle and take a position across from the litter. The front of the litter is then handed to them across the object.

Yes: ❑ Reteach: ❑ Return: ❑ Instructor initials: ________

Step 2: As the litter is passed forward, the two EMTs in the rear move forward to take position beyond the obstacle. All EMTs remain standing with feet firmly planted as the litter is passed. Once the litter is beyond and clear of the obstacle, all EMTs turn and face forward. The EMTs may then move forward together as a unit.

Yes: ❑ Reteach: ❑ Return: ❑ Instructor initials: ________

Chapter 11 Skill Sheet

Student Name ________________________________ Date ________________

Skill 11-17: The Bedroll

Equipment Needed:

1. Appropriate PPE
2. Stretcher, blanket, sheet, pillow, pillowcase

Yes: ❑ Reteach: ❑ Return: ❑ Instructor initials: ________

Step 1: The first EMT lays the blanket centered onto the stretcher, then the sheet on top of that.

Yes: ❑ Reteach: ❑ Return: ❑ Instructor initials: ________

Step 2: The first and second EMT grasp one half of the linen and fold it in half, creating a collar. Repeat with the other side. To open the bedroll, the EMTs simply grasp the collars and fold the edges.

Yes: ❑ Reteach: ❑ Return: ❑ Instructor initials: ________

Step 3: With the patient lying supine, the EMTs can fold the upper edge over the patient's head, then secure the edge with the lower edge. The pillow should then be placed behind the head, outside the linen.

Yes: ❑ Reteach: ❑ Return: ❑ Instructor initials: ________

Chapter 11 Skill Sheet

Student Name ______________________________ Date ________________

Skill 11-18: The Carry Transfer

Equipment Needed:

1. Appropriate PPE
2. Two stretchers, gurneys

Yes: ❑ Reteach: ❑ Return: ❑ Instructor initials: ________

Step 1: The first stretcher is placed with the patient's head at the foot of the other stretcher at a 90-degree angle.

Yes: ❑ Reteach: ❑ Return: ❑ Instructor initials: ________

Step 2: The two EMTs stand on the side of patient. The first EMT places one arm under the patient's head and neck and the other arm under the shoulders. The second EMT places his arms under the patient's lower back and buttocks.

Yes: ❑ Reteach: ❑ Return: ❑ Instructor initials: ________

Step 3: Simultaneously, the two EMTs hoist the patient to their chest. Shuffling sideways, the two EMTs move the patient to the awaiting stretcher.

Yes: ❑ Reteach: ❑ Return: ❑ Instructor initials: ________

Step 4: The patient is then gently laid onto the stretcher. The EMT should be sure that all stretcher straps are attached before moving the patient.

Yes: ❑ Reteach: ❑ Return: ❑ Instructor initials: ________

Chapter 11 Skill Sheet

Student Name ______________________________ Date ______________

Skill 11-19: The Draw Sheet Transfer

Equipment Needed:

1. Appropriate PPE
2. Two stretchers, draw sheet or bed linen

Yes: ❑ Reteach: ❑ Return: ❑ Instructor initials: ________

Step 1: The two stretchers are placed side by side. The EMT should be sure that the stretcher brakes are engaged before moving the patient. Any side rails present will have to be lowered.

Yes: ❑ Reteach: ❑ Return: ❑ Instructor initials: ________

Step 2: Two EMTs are on the one open side of both stretchers. Rolling the edge of the draw sheet or bed linen into a collar, the EMTs grab a firm purchase. (It is a good practice to have the two teams of EMTs pull vigorously against each other to test the strength of the sheet.)

Yes: ❑ Reteach: ❑ Return: ❑ Instructor initials: ________

Step 3: Simultaneously, the four EMTs slide the patient from one stretcher to the other in one fluid motion.

Yes: ❑ Reteach: ❑ Return: ❑ Instructor initials: ________

Step 4: Once the patient is on the new stretcher, the side rails should be replaced.

Yes: ❑ Reteach: ❑ Return: ❑ Instructor initials: ________

CHAPTER 12
Scene Size-Up

This chapter stresses those protective behaviors an EMT should practice while on-scene.

Completion: Complete the following sentences using the Key Terms in Chapter 12 of the textbook.

1. The ____________________ ____________________ is the first radio report of the scene conditions.

2. The feeling that there is an increased likelihood of injury is based on a ____________________ ____________________ of ____________________.

3. A device intended to produce death is a(n) ____________________ ____________________, while one capable of death or serious harm in certain circumstances is a(n) ____________________ ____________________.

4. The ____________________ divides hazardous areas from nonhazardous areas. A barrier that protects EMTs and permits them to work is a(n) ____________________ ____________________.

5. A scene ____________________ must be done to determine if any hazards are on-scene. Emergency vehicles can then be ____________________ safely in a specific place.

Identification: For each area of the vehicle, write down information that is relevant to the EMT's damage survey.

1. bumpers ____
2. fenders ____
3. body ____
4. windshield ____
5. passenger compartment ____
6. underneath ____

Identification: Place an X in front of those actions that an EMT should do to assist in vehicle stabilization.

_____ Enter a car sitting on its roof

_____ Take the transmission out of drive

_____ Turn off the engine

_____ Chock the wheels

_____ Close windows

_____ Cut seat belts

_____ Engage parking brake

True or False: Read each statement and decide if it is true or false. Place a T or F on the line before each statement.

1. _____ Upon arrival, the ambulance should be parked right next to the scene to prevent the crew from injuring themselves carrying heavy equipment.
2. _____ The EMT should treat all downed wires as dangerous.
3. _____ The single greatest danger to the EMT at a car crash is leaking fluids.
4. _____ OSHA requires all emergency vehicles to have at least one blue light.
5. _____ The safest place for an ambulance is ahead of the motor vehicle collision.
6. _____ If possible, place the ambulance in the direction of travel to the hospital.

7. ____ Flares are designed to prevent inadvertent ignition of spilled fluids.
8. ____ On a 40 mph straightaway, place the first flare 160 feet from the crash.
9. ____ A starred windshield results from something striking it at a specific point.
10. ____ EMTs provide treatment to multiple patients according to a sorting plan.

Correcting: Rewrite each of the following as a correct statement by replacing or deleting the underlined words.

1. On the scene of a major incident, the safety officer functions as a member of the <u>operations staff</u>.
2. Stopping the emergency vehicle a safe distance from the scene is called <u>scene survey</u>.
3. Courts have upheld the idea that an EMT <u>cannot refuse</u> to enter a dangerous situation.
4. To place flares on a curve, <u>add two times the radius of the curve</u> to the distance listed on the chart.

Short Answer: Based on each damage descriptor, list the probable point of patient impact.

1. Broken rearview mirror

2. Bent steering wheel

3. Broken dash

4. Seat knocked off pedestal

5. Locked seat belt

Critical Thinking 1: Read the following scenario and then answer the questions.

Dan and Deborah were called to a gas station following the inadvertent release of dry chemicals from an overhead fire extinguisher system. Once there, they found 10 people on the scene, all covered with a white powder. One patron had tripped over the gas can that he was filling, spilling the liquid onto the ground. Another was speaking loudly on a cell phone detailing the reasons she would be late for a meeting.

What scene hazards are present here?

Critical Thinking 2: Read the following scenario and then answer the questions.

Jorge and Marrissa answered a call at the terminus of a high-speed highway. A driver, not paying attention to the END HIGHWAY signs, struck two other cars, resulting in great damage and the leaking of fluids. A police officer has set out flares but has not closed down the highway.

What scene hazards are present here?

Critical Thinking 3: Read the following scenario and then answer the questions.

Dory and Chris have answered a call at a small out-of-the-way house. While the rest of the area has become suburbanized with new homes and immaculate lawns, this area has remained just as it was 60 years ago—small truck farms with some agricultural animals. There are no sidewalks and no street lights. The home is run-down but appears clean. A sign inside the front door reads, "Home protected by Smith and Wesson."

What scene hazards are present here?

Chapter 12 Skill Sheet

Student Name ______________________________ Date ________________

Skill 12-1: Lighting a Road Flare

Equipment Needed:

1. Road flare
2. Helmet with eye shield
3. Gloves
4. Turnout coat

Yes: ❑ Reteach: ❑ Return: ❑ Instructor initials: ________

Step 1: The EMT should put on eye protection and gloves. (It is preferable for the EMT to wear a turnout coat as well.)

Yes: ❑ Reteach: ❑ Return: ❑ Instructor initials: ________

Step 2: The EMT holds the flare 6 inches below the head, then removes the striker from the end of the flare.

Yes: ❑ Reteach: ❑ Return: ❑ Instructor initials: ________

Step 3: The EMT briskly strikes the striker against the flare's igniter while aiming it away from his body.

Yes: ❑ Reteach: ❑ Return: ❑ Instructor initials: ________

Step 4: The EMT keeps the lit flare away from his body and places it on the ground.

Yes: ❑ Reteach: ❑ Return: ❑ Instructor initials: ________

Chapter 12 Skill Sheet

Student Name ______________________________ Date ________________

Skill 12-2: Vehicle Stabilization

Equipment Needed:

1. Flashlight
2. Turnout gear
3. Helmet

Yes: ❑ Reteach: ❑ Return: ❑ Instructor initials: ________

Step 1: The first EMT circles the car starting from the driver's side. The EMT advises the patient to sit still for a minute. The EMT checks for vehicle damage.

Yes: ❑ Reteach: ❑ Return: ❑ Instructor initials: ________

Step 2: The second EMT circles the car from the opposite side. The EMT checks for hazards above and underneath the car.

Yes: ❑ Reteach: ❑ Return: ❑ Instructor initials: ________

Step 3: After the second EMT calls "all clear," the first EMT enters the passenger side and stabilizes the patient's head.

Yes: ❑ Reteach: ❑ Return: ❑ Instructor initials: ________

Step 4: The first EMT then reaches in and checks to see that the car is in park.

Yes: ❑ Reteach: ❑ Return: ❑ Instructor initials: ________

Step 5: The EMT confirms the car is turned off. The EMT checks for electric locks, windows, and seats first.

Yes: ❑ Reteach: ❑ Return: ❑ Instructor initials: ________

Step 6: The EMT confirms that the car's emergency brake is engaged.

Yes: ❑ Reteach: ❑ Return: ❑ Instructor initials: ________

CHAPTER 13
Initial Assessment

It is important for the EMT-B to attempt to perform the initial assessment the same way each time. Of course, it will vary slightly depending upon the patient situation, but the order of priorities must always remain the same. This chapter covers the recommended method of completing an initial assessment.

Identification: Place a checkmark in front of those items that should be assessed or found on an initial assessment.

_____ an injured, deformed leg

_____ vomit in the mouth

_____ history of a heart attack

_____ crepitus over the neck and chest

_____ a bone deformed in the arm

_____ gives a complete medical history

_____ use of cocaine

_____ a stab wound to the chest

_____ absent radial pulse

_____ allergy to penicillin

_____ snoring respirations

_____ blood-soaked jeans

_____ breakfast last eaten

_____ tenderness of chest wall

Identification: Decide if each patient is alert, verbal, responsive to pain, or unresponsive. Place the correct letter—A, V, P, or U—on the line before each description.

1. _____ The patient asks appropriate questions.
2. _____ There is no movement at all when a woman's skin is pinched.
3. _____ A man moans "uh huh" if spoken to loudly.
4. _____ The patient moves only if pressure is applied to her fingernail.
5. _____ A child watches where Mom and Dad go.
6. _____ A woman speaks rapidly to the EMT-B in a foreign language.
7. _____ The patient appears to go to sleep when the EMT-B stops talking.
8. _____ A child opens her eyes when spoken to in a loud voice.
9. _____ A patient opens her eyes only when the shoulder is pinched.

Sorting: Place the following descriptions under the correct heading of patent airway or nonpatent airway.

snoring	broken teeth in mouth	very bloody nose
speaking clearly	stridor	quiet breathing
drooling	vomitus	good chest rise
unresponsive	infant unable to cry	alert and oriented

Patent	**Nonpatent**

True or False: Read each statement and decide if it is true or false. Place T or F on the line before each statement.

1. _____ Breathing is checked after the pulse.
2. _____ To adequately check breathing, look, listen, and feel.
3. _____ An adequate respiratory rate for an adult is between 10 and 28 breaths per minute.
4. _____ Chest injuries may impair breathing adequacy.
5. _____ Open chest wounds impede adequate lung expansion.
6. _____ Wheezing may indicate a partial airway obstruction.
7. _____ Subcutaneous air feels like a sponge.
8. _____ Check for a pulse on an infant at the radius.
9. _____ When checking a pulse in a hypothermic patient, count for one full minute.
10. _____ All bleeding should be immediately controlled.
11. _____ Capillary refill is a good indicator of perfusion in a 2-year-old.

Definitions: Write the definitions of the following terms.

1. alert ______________________________
2. crepitus ______________________________
3. sternal rub ______________________________
4. flail chest ______________________________
5. paradoxical motion ______________________________
6. AVPU ______________________________
7. ABCs ______________________________
8. unresponsive ______________________________

Short Answer: Read each question. Think about the information presented in your text, and then answer each question with one or two sentences.

1. What does the "look test" tell the EMT?

2. During the B step of the initial assessment, the EMT finds that the patient is breathing. What other information must he obtain before he moves on in his assessment?

3. What type(s) of bleeding must be controlled during the initial assessment?

Identification: Read each patient presentation and determine if the patient is high or low priority. Place the word "high" or "low" on the line in front of each presentation.

1. __________ Looks ill
2. __________ Has a swollen deformed arm

3. ___________ Is complaining of some dizziness
4. ___________ Verbally responds but doesn't follow commands
5. ___________ Back pain after a motor vehicle collision
6. ___________ Respiratory rate 34 and shallow
7. ___________ Excessive bleeding from a leg wound
8. ___________ Anxious, rapid breathing and pulse
9. ___________ Normal childbirth

Critical Thinking 1: Read the scenario and then answer the questions.

Jeff and Makenzi were called to the dorm room of a young male patient who would not wake up. His buddies said he had spent the night cramming for an exam and when they went to get him today, they couldn't get him to wake up.

The EMT-Bs found a young man lying supine on the floor of his dorm room. His skin was very pale and he didn't answer when his name was called.

1. Is there a potentially life-threatening condition present? If so, what is it?

2. Based on the limited information available, what should the EMT-Bs anticipate with regard to the airway?

3. What priority would you assign to this patient?

Critical Thinking 2: Read the scenario and then answer the questions.

Fran and Eric answered a call to the local nursing home for a patient not feeling well. Upon their arrival, they found Mr. Edgars sitting at the end of his bed. He told the EMT-Bs that his stomach had been upset for two days and he didn't feel much like eating. He also said he hadn't vomited, just that he felt "yecchy."

1. Is there a potentially life-threatening condition present? If so, what is it?

2. Based on the limited information available, what do the EMT-Bs know about Mr. Edgars airway?

3. What priority would you assign to this patient?

Critical Thinking 3: Read the scenario and then answer the questions.

Dean and Donny were dispatched to a woman ready to give birth. Upon their arrival, they found Mrs. Green lying on her couch. She looked pale and sweaty. There was an excessive amount of blood present on her clothing and she complained of unbearable pain.

1. Is there a potentially life-threatening condition present? If so, what is it?

2. Based on the limited information available, what should the EMT-Bs anticipate with regard to perfusion?

3. What priority would you assign to this patient?

Chapter 13 Skill Sheet

Student Name ______________________________ Date ________________

Skill 13-1: The Initial Assessment

Equipment Needed:

1. Appropriate PPE
2. Stethoscope
3. Scissors
4. Airway management equipment

Yes: ❑ Reteach: ❑ Return: ❑ Instructor initials: ________

Step 1: The EMT surveys the scene for safety hazards as well as any potential mechanism of injury. Needed personal protective equipment should be donned now.

Yes: ❑ Reteach: ❑ Return: ❑ Instructor initials: ________

Step 2: The EMT forms a general impression of the scene; deciding, for example, whether it is trauma or medical.

Yes: ❑ Reteach: ❑ Return: ❑ Instructor initials: ________

Step 3: The EMT next determines the patient's mental status on the AVPU scale. If the scene is trauma, another EMT immediately takes head stabilization first.

Yes: ❑ Reteach: ❑ Return: ❑ Instructor initials: ________

Step 4: The EMT assesses and manages the airway as needed.

Yes: ❑ Reteach: ❑ Return: ❑ Instructor initials: ________

Step 5: Next, the EMT assesses and manages breathing.

Yes: ❑ Reteach: ❑ Return: ❑ Instructor initials: ________

Step 6: Finally, the EMT assesses and manages circulation. If the patient is high priority, transportation should be initiated immediately.

Yes: ❑ Reteach: ❑ Return: ❑ Instructor initials: ________

CHAPTER 14 Focused History and Physical Examination of the Trauma Patient

Once the initial assessment is complete and no life threats found, the EMT-B completes the focused history and physical exam.

Word Scramble: Unscramble the following terms.

1. nobarsia ______________________________
2. nubr ______________________________
3. ustnncooi ______________________________
4. ytorfmied ______________________________
5. gradguin ______________________________
6. craatilnoe ______________________________
7. uuptcner ______________________________
8. liwsnelg ______________________________
9. trened ______________________________
10. tiprecsu ______________________________

True or False: Read each statement and decide if it is true or false. Place T or F on the line before each statement.

1. _____ It is easy to determine if a patient has a medical or a trauma problem.
2. _____ All patients are trauma until proven otherwise.
3. _____ The medical history is gathered after the trauma physical exam.
4. _____ The rapid trauma exam is used to find injuries not initially evident.
5. _____ In minor trauma, the EMT-B performs a focused trauma exam.
6. _____ All unconscious patients should have a rapid trauma exam.
7. _____ Gruesome bone injuries require immediate attention.
8. _____ All trauma patients need spinal immobilization.
9. _____ The initial assessment is performed only once.
10. _____ A rapid trauma exam begins at the head and progresses to the feet.

Listing: List six principles for conducting a physical exam.

1. ____
2. ____
3. ____
4. ____
5. ____
6. ____

Identification: Place a checkmark in front of the serious trauma by mechanisms.

_____ Vehicle rollover with unrestrained patient

_____ Fall of 10 feet

_____ Death of another occupant in the vehicle

_____ Farm trauma

_____ Vehicle-pedestrian accident

_____ Twenty inches of front-end damage

_____ Ejection

_____ Motorcycle accident

_____ Crash speed of 20 mph or greater

Ordering: Put the steps for completing a rapid trauma exam in order by placing the numeral 1 before the first step, 2 before the second, and so on.

_____ Obtain baseline vitals signs

_____ Document

_____ Size-up/scene safety

_____ Obtain a SAMPLE history

_____ Complete an initial assessment, including spinal precautions

_____ Consider ALS

_____ Complete a rapid trauma assessment

Completion: Write out the word suggested by each letter of the acronym DCAP-BTLS. Explain what each word means.

D

C

A

P

B

T

L

S

What does this acronym remind the EMT-B to do?

Critical Thinking 1: Read the scenario and then answer the questions.

A teenager trips on a high curb and injures his right ankle. There is no fall and no loss of consciousness.

1. Would this be considered major or minor trauma according to the table of serious mechanisms?

2. From your textbook, list the exams that will be performed.

Critical Thinking 2: Read the scenario and then answer the questions.

A young man is involved in a rollover accident on the interstate.

1. Would this be considered major or minor trauma according to the table of serious mechanisms?

2. From your textbook, list the exams that will be performed.

Critical Thinking 3: Read the scenario and then answer the questions.

A roofer falls from a church steeple.

1. Would this be considered major or minor trauma according to the table of serious mechanisms?

2. From your textbook, list the exams that will be performed.

Critical Thinking 4: Read the scenario and then answer the questions.

A woman is struck by the side of a car just as the car is leaving a stoplight.

1. Would this be considered major or minor trauma according to the table of serious mechanisms?

2. From your textbook, list the exams that will be performed.

Critical Thinking 5: Read the scenario and then answer the questions.

A skateboarder falls down six steps at the public library. There is no loss of consciousness.

1. Would this be considered major or minor trauma according to the table of serious mechanisms?

2. From your textbook, list the exams that will be performed.

Chapter 14 Skill Sheet

Student Name ______________________________ Date ________________

Skill 14-1: Rapid Trauma Assessment

Equipment Needed:

1. Appropriate PPE
2. Stethoscope
3. Blood pressure cuff
4. Scissors
5. Cervical collars

Yes: ❑ Reteach: ❑ Return: ❑ Instructor initials: ________

Step 1: After completing an appropriate scene size-up and initial assessment, the EMT performs a rapid trauma assessment on the trauma patient with a significant mechanism of injury. Manual head stabilization is maintained for the duration of the rapid trauma assessment.

Yes: ❑ Reteach: ❑ Return: ❑ Instructor initials: ________

Step 2: The EMT should consider a request for ALS backup and determine the transport priority. Most seriously injured trauma patients are en route to the hospital while the rapid trauma assessment is being done.

Yes: ❑ Reteach: ❑ Return: ❑ Instructor initials: ________

Step 3: The EMT next assesses the head by careful inspection and palpation for signs of injury. Deformities, contusions, abrasions, punctures/penetrations, burns, tenderness, lacerations, or swelling should be noted. Moving in a methodical fashion, the EMT next inspects and palpates the neck.

Yes: ❑ Reteach: ❑ Return: ❑ Instructor initials: ________

Step 4: The EMT next looks, listens, and feels the chest to assess for presence of any signs of injury. Breath sounds are carefully assessed at the apices and bases. Presence and equality of air movement is noted.

Yes: ❑ Reteach: ❑ Return: ❑ Instructor initials: ________

Step 5: The abdominal assessment includes looking and feeling for any signs of injury. The pelvis is visually inspected, then gently compressed downward and inward in order to find any signs of injury.

Yes: ❑ Reteach: ❑ Return: ❑ Instructor initials: ________

(continues)

Chapter 14 Skill Sheet

Skill 14-1: *Continued*

Step 6: After rolling the patient to the side using a logroll technique and maintaining spinal immobilization, the EMT inspects and palpates the back and buttocks to find signs of injury.

Yes: ❑ Reteach: ❑ Return: ❑ Instructor initials: ________

Step 7: After completing the rapid trauma assessment, a complete baseline set of vital signs must be taken.

Yes: ❑ Reteach: ❑ Return: ❑ Instructor initials: ________

Step 8: A SAMPLE history is elicited. Bystanders may provide information if the patient is unconscious. Transport should have been initiated by this point.

Yes: ❑ Reteach: ❑ Return: ❑ Instructor initials: ________

Chapter 14 Skill Sheet

Student Name ______________________ Date ____________

Skill 14-2: Focused Trauma Assessment

Equipment Needed:

1. Stethoscope
2. Blood pressure cuff
3. Assortment of cervical collars

Yes: ❑ Reteach: ❑ Return: ❑ Instructor initials: ________

Step 1: The EMT considers the mechanism of injury. Depending on the mechanism of injury, the EMT decides whether to perform a rapid trauma assessment or a focused physical examination.

Yes: ❑ Reteach: ❑ Return: ❑ Instructor initials: ________

Step 2: The EMT next determines the chief complaint.

Yes: ❑ Reteach: ❑ Return: ❑ Instructor initials: ________

Step 3: The EMT performs a focused examination specific to the injury.

Yes: ❑ Reteach: ❑ Return: ❑ Instructor initials: ________

Step 4: The EMT then obtains baseline vital signs.

Yes: ❑ Reteach: ❑ Return: ❑ Instructor initials: ________

Step 5: The EMT completes the assessment with a SAMPLE history.

Yes: ❑ Reteach: ❑ Return: ❑ Instructor initials: ________

CHAPTER 15
Detailed Physical Examination

The detailed physical exam is a patient-specific and injury-specific examination. It is performed on patients who have significant injuries or a significant mechanism of injury.

Matching: Match each word or term with its definition.

1. _____ Battle's sign
2. _____ cerebrospinal fluid
3. _____ hyphema
4. _____ PERRL
5. _____ raccoon eyes
6. _____ seat belt sign
7. _____ PMS
8. _____ urinary incontinence

a. bruising behind the ears
b. description of normal pupils
c. a red mark left by a car restraint device
d. pulses, motor, sensory
e. blood in the anterior chamber of the eye
f. fluid that bathes the spinal cord and brain
g. loss of control of the bladder
h. bruising around the eyes

True or False: Read each statement and decide if it is true or false. Place T or F on the line before each statement.

1. _____ Compression/flexion of the pelvis is not indicated if a pelvic injury is already suspected.
2. _____ The detailed physical exam is focused on the complaint only.
3. _____ The detailed physical exam is performed on patients with serious injuries.
4. _____ Use DCAP-BTLS as the mnemonic for the detailed physical exam.
5. _____ Apply direct pressure to stop the flow of CSF from the nose or ears.
6. _____ In the halo test, blood will spread out and around the CSF.
7. _____ Bruising behind the ears may indicate a fracture at the base of the skull.
8. _____ Bruising around the eyes is indicative of a temporal skull fracture.
9. _____ Unequal pupils always indicate a head injury.
10. _____ Loose dentures should be removed.

Ordering: Place a 1 before the action that should be completed first, a 2 in front of the next action, and so on.

_____ Rapid trauma exam

_____ First impression

_____ Scene survey/size-up

_____ Detailed exam

_____ Initial exam

Listing: List the specific things that should be assessed in each region.

skull ______

ears ______

eyes ______

face ______

nose ______

mouth ______

neck ______

chest ______

abdomen ______

extremities ______

Critical Thinking 1: Read the scenario and then answer the questions.

Tom and Howard answered to a call at a construction site. A construction worker had fallen 10 feet from scaffolding to a sandy surface. First responders indicated that the worker had probably suffered a head injury.

1. What injuries should the EMTs discover in the initial exam?

2. What injuries should the EMTs discover in the detailed physical exam that would lead to the conclusion of a head injury?

Critical Thinking 2: Read the scenario and then answer the questions.

Georgette and Christopher were on their way to quarters when they came upon a motor vehicle collision. The primary ambulance crew had triaged patients, and Georgette and Chris were assigned to care for a 60-year-old man who was a restrained passenger in a vehicle that was struck head on. Mr. Smith complained of feeling shaken but otherwise unhurt. The car suffered extensive front-end damage. The initial assessment showed no life threats. Rapid trauma exam showed a reddened area across the abdomen and right shoulder. No other injuries were noted. While the EMTs were completing the detailed exam, the patient complained that he felt anxious and thirsty and that his heart was racing.

1. What further injuries can be expected on the detailed physical exam?

2. What problem might explain the increased heart rate, change in mental status, and injuries noted on the detailed exam?

Chapter 15 Skill Sheet

Student Name ______________________________ Date ________________

Skill 15-1: Detailed Physical Examination

Equipment Needed:

1. Penlight
2. Stethoscope
3. Blood pressure cuff
4. Scissors

Yes: ❑ Reteach: ❑ Return: ❑ Instructor initials: ________

Step 1: Start at the top of the head and assess the scalp and the face for DCAP-BTLS.

Yes: ❑ Reteach: ❑ Return: ❑ Instructor initials: ________

Step 2: Next, assess the ears, nose, and throat, noting any bleeding or drainage of fluids, as well as jugular venous distention or displacement of the trachea.

Yes: ❑ Reteach: ❑ Return: ❑ Instructor initials: ________

Step 3: Then, proceed to looking, listening, and feeling the chest wall for injury, including crepitus and paradoxical motion.

Yes: ❑ Reteach: ❑ Return: ❑ Instructor initials: ________

Step 4: Turning next to the abdomen and the pelvis, assess for DCAP-BTLS. Assessment of the pelvis should include gentle pressure inward on the hips to check for a hip fracture.

Yes: ❑ Reteach: ❑ Return: ❑ Instructor initials: ________

Step 5: Then, assess the extremities for pulses, movement, and sensation, as well as DCAP-BTLS.

Yes: ❑ Reteach: ❑ Return: ❑ Instructor initials: ________

Step 6: After checking as much of the posterior as possible, obtain another set of vital signs.

Yes: ❑ Reteach: ❑ Return: ❑ Instructor initials: ________

CHAPTER 16 Focused History and Physical Examination of the Medical Patient

The priorities of a patient suffering from a medical illness are somewhat different than the patient suffering from a trauma. These priorities change based on whether the medical patient is awake and responsive or unresponsive.

Sorting: Place the information into its correct category.

headache	asthma attack one week ago	eczema
hives with penicillin	wheezing after eating nuts	ate breakfast
Ventolin q6 hours	aspirin daily	cleaning with bleach
asthma	Theo-Dur QID	shortness of breath

S	A	M	P	L	E

Ordering: Place in order of completion for a responsive medical patient.

_____ Ongoing assessment

_____ Chief complaint

_____ SAMPLE

_____ Baseline vital signs

_____ OPQRST

_____ Initial assessment

_____ Treat and transport

_____ Focused physical exam

Ordering: Place in order of completion for an unresponsive medical patient.

_____ SAMPLE history

_____ Initial assessment

_____ Treat and transport

_____ Baseline vital signs

_____ Rapid physical exam

_____ Ongoing assessment

Short Answer: For each patient, decide which assessment format you will use.

1. ______________________________ Unconscious, lying in bed
2. ______________________________ Awake, crying, cut hand on glass
3. ______________________________ Unconscious at base of ladder

4. ______________________ Walked into station complaining of a headache
5. ______________________ Superficial stab wound to thigh
6. ______________________ Gunshot wound to the chest
7. ______________________ Severe cough and fever
8. ______________________ Not responding after eating cookies
9. ______________________ Abdominal pain after car crash
10. ______________________ Abdominal pain and vomiting after dinner

Definitions: Write the definition of the following terms.

1. chief complaint ______________________
2. focused physical exam ______________________
3. medic alert bracelet ______________________
4. ongoing assessment ______________________
5. on-line medical control ______________________
6. OPQRST ______________________
7. SAMPLE ______________________
8. vial of life ______________________

True or False: Read each statement and decide if it is true or false. Place T or F on the line before each statement.

1. _____ The history of the present illness in a medical patient is the equivalent of the mechanism of injury for the trauma patient.
2. _____ The chief complaint is determined by the EMT after the focused exam is completed.
3. _____ The history should guide the EMT in focusing the physical exam.
4. _____ Abnormal vital signs should prompt the EMT to initiate immediate transport.
5. _____ The rapid physical exam for the medical patient is conducted in the same way as for the trauma patient.
6. _____ Transport should always be initiated before the rapid trauma exam.
7. _____ If an EMT has a question about providing a treatment, she should arrange an ALS intercept.
8. _____ Contact with the receiving facility should include the nature of the patient's problem.
9. _____ All medical patients are managed in the same way.

Critical Thinking 1: Read the scenario and then answer the questions.

Steve and Donna were assessing an unresponsive patient found in bed by family members.

1. Name at least three ways to obtain information on this patient.

2. When would transport be initiated for this patient?

Critical Thinking 2: Read the scenario and then answer the question.

Dana and Greg were attending to Mrs. Fleming, who called complaining of a headache. As the EMTs were obtaining the SAMPLE history, Mrs. Fleming also told them about an upset stomach, pain in both legs, dizziness, and lack of appetite.

1. What is the chief complaint?

Chapter 16 Skill Sheet

Student Name ______________________________ Date ________________

Skill 16-1: Focused Medical Assessment—Responsive Medical Patient

Equipment Needed:

1. Penlight
2. Stethoscope
3. Blood pressure cuff
4. Scissors

Yes: ❑ Reteach: ❑ Return: ❑ Instructor initials: ________

Step 1: Obtain a chief complaint and a history of the present illness, using the OPQRST format when appropriate.

Yes: ❑ Reteach: ❑ Return: ❑ Instructor initials: ________

Step 2: After obtaining the history of the present illness, take the patient's SAMPLE history.

Yes: ❑ Reteach: ❑ Return: ❑ Instructor initials: ________

Step 3: On the basis of the patient's chief complaint, perform a focused physical examination of the affected area. After the physical examination, obtain a baseline set of vital signs.

Yes: ❑ Reteach: ❑ Return: ❑ Instructor initials: ________

Step 4: It may be necessary to assist the patient with his medications or transport the patient to the hospital. An ongoing assessment should be continued en route to the hospital.

Yes: ❑ Reteach: ❑ Return: ❑ Instructor initials: ________

Chapter 16 Skill Sheet

Student Name ______________________________ Date ________________

Skill 16-2: Rapid Medical Examination—Unresponsive Medical Patient

Equipment Needed:

1. Penlight
2. Stethoscope
3. Blood pressure cuff
4. Scissors

Yes: ❑ Reteach: ❑ Return: ❑ Instructor initials: ________

Step 1: Quickly perform an initial assessment.

Yes: ❑ Reteach: ❑ Return: ❑ Instructor initials: ________

Step 2: Proceed to a rapid physical examination of the patient.

Yes: ❑ Reteach: ❑ Return: ❑ Instructor initials: ________

Step 3: As soon as is practical, a baseline set of vital signs is obtained as well.

Yes: ❑ Reteach: ❑ Return: ❑ Instructor initials: ________

Step 4: Bystanders or family members should be questioned about the patient's illness and past medical history.

Yes: ❑ Reteach: ❑ Return: ❑ Instructor initials: ________

Step 5: Transport the patient as soon as possible.

Yes: ❑ Reteach: ❑ Return: ❑ Instructor initials: ________

Step 6: En route to the hospital, contact medical control and consider meeting with ALS.

Yes: ❑ Reteach: ❑ Return: ❑ Instructor initials: ________

CHAPTER 17
The Ongoing Assessment

The EMT is responsible for observing and caring for the patient until arrival at the hospital, where care will be turned over to the hospital staff.

Short Answer: Read each question. Think about the information presented in your text, and then answer each question with one or two sentences.

1. State two reasons for performing the ongoing assessment.

2. When is the ongoing assessment conducted?

Identification: Place an X next to those items evaluated in the ongoing assessment.

_____	mental status	_____	history
_____	airway	_____	pulses
_____	SAMPLE	_____	effectiveness of meds
_____	baseline vital signs	_____	home safety
_____	breathing	_____	abrasions to forearms
_____	empty oxygen tank	_____	bleeding
_____	pulse oximetry	_____	pulse, respirations, BP
_____	distal pulses		

Critical Thinking: Locate the trends in each scenario, and then indicate whether the patient's condition (priority) has changed.

1. Ongoing assessment shows that the pulse rate has increased by 20 beats per minute, and the patient is now extremely anxious.

2. The respiratory rate has dropped from 28 breaths per minute to 20 breaths per minute. The patient can now say five words per breath as opposed to two words per breath.

3. The patient had been answering questions appropriately. Now she is increasingly sleepy and gives only one-word answers.

Chapter 17 Skill Sheet

Student Name ______________________________ Date _______________

Skill 17-1: Ongoing Assessment

Equipment Needed:

1. Penlight
2. Stethoscope
3. Blood pressure cuff

Yes: ❑ Reteach: ❑ Return: ❑ Instructor initials: ________

Step 1: While en route to the hospital, repeat the initial assessment, reassessing the patient's mental status using the AVPU scale and monitoring the airway.

Yes: ❑ Reteach: ❑ Return: ❑ Instructor initials: ________

Step 2: The patient's breathing must be reassessed for rate and quality, and lung sounds must be monitored.

Yes: ❑ Reteach: ❑ Return: ❑ Instructor initials: ________

Step 3: Reassess the patient's circulatory status, including skin temperature, and note any additional bleeding.

Yes: ❑ Reteach: ❑ Return: ❑ Instructor initials: ________

Step 4: After mentally reviewing the patient's priorities, reassess vital signs and repeat a physical examination as needed.

Yes: ❑ Reteach: ❑ Return: ❑ Instructor initials: ________

Step 5: Recheck the interventions, such as oxygen tank pressures.

Yes: ❑ Reteach: ❑ Return: ❑ Instructor initials: ________

CHAPTER 18
Radio

EMTs need a rudimentary understanding of communication systems and how to operate them. These systems are a part of the daily life of an EMT.

Definitions: Write the definitions of the following terms.

1. base station ____________________
2. communications center ____________________
3. communications specialist ____________________
4. med channel ____________________
5. tactical channel ____________________
6. trunked line ____________________

Matching: Match each word or term with its definition.

1.	_____	affirmative	a.	multiple users on one frequency
2.	_____	digital technology	b.	radio code, replacing words
3.	_____	FM radio	c.	channel used to call a specific agency or hospital
4.	_____	echo technique	d.	a radio that can transmit or receive but not at the same time
5.	_____	negative	e.	a wave speed measurement
6.	_____	channel crowding	f.	very high frequency
7.	_____	scanner	g.	term meaning "yes"
8.	_____	UHF	h.	radio that alters the speed of a wave
9.	_____	special codes	i.	picks up a signal and boosts it
10.	_____	hailing frequency	j.	also known as a channel
11.	_____	VHF	k.	ultra high frequency
12.	_____	repeater	l.	a device permitting the public to listen to EMS channels
13.	_____	megahertz	m.	term meaning "no"
14.	_____	frequency	n.	repetition to confirm what was said
15.	_____	simplex	o.	conversion into digitally coded signals

Listing: List the six roles of a communications specialist.

1.
2.
3.

4.

5.

6.

Identification: Place the name of the radio system component on the line before each description.

1. ____________________ Wireless electronic device permitting transmission of messages to radio receivers
2. ____________________ Large powerful radio located at a stationary site
3. ____________________ Radio located inside a vehicle
4. ____________________ Receiver that picks up the signal and boosts it
5. ____________________ Handheld radio
6. ____________________ Radio that either receives or transmits, but not both at same time
7. ____________________ Radio similar in nature to a phone

Sorting: Read the information below. If the information should be part of an alert report, mark A. If it is part of a consultation report, mark C. If it is part of both reports, mark B.

_____ unit identifier

_____ ETA

_____ mental status

_____ treatments in progress

_____ exam findings

_____ age/gender

_____ chief complaint

_____ vital signs

_____ SAMPLE

_____ changes after treatments

Short Answer: Read each question. Think about the information presented in your text, and then answer each question with one or two sentences.

1. How do communications specialists protect the public during an EMS call?

2. Name three ways in which communications specialists reduce injury or death of patients who call for EMS assistance.

3. Why are communications specialists called the "first first responders"?

4. Describe the role of the FCC in EMS communications.

Critical Thinking: Read the following scenario and write both an alert report and a consultation report.

ARS unit 1, a BLS response vehicle, arrived at the scene of a 70-year-old woman living in a retirement home. Her neighbors reported that she "wasn't acting herself" that day. The woman just said her head hurt a lot. She had participated in card games the evening before and seemed OK. It was only today that anyone noticed a change. Medicines located on the kitchen counter included pills for high blood pressure, eye drops for glaucoma, and a daily aspirin.

The woman was awake but couldn't seem to get simple answers straight. She also kept complaining of her headache. Initial and focused exams showed no signs of bleeding or injury. Lung sounds were clear. Respirations were 16 per minute and non-labored. Her pulse was strong at the wrist and 64 per minute and regular. BP was 198/98. There was a noticeable droop to her mouth as she tried to smile, and her left-hand grasp was much weaker than the right.

The EMTs placed her onto the stretcher, began high-flow oxygen, and requested an ALS intercept. They hoped to meet up with the ALS within 10 minutes. It would take them 20 minutes to arrive at the hospital.

CHAPTER 19
Report

Giving a patient report offers two health care professionals an opportunity to focus on one patient and exchange observations, records, and physical findings.

Definitions: Give an example of each of the following terms.

1. abandonment ____
2. confidentiality ____
3. repetitive persistence ____
4. verbal report ____

Listing: List the three rights of effective interpersonal communications.

1.
2.
3.

Critical Thinking 1: Read the scenario and then answer the questions.

Jeff and Suzanne arrived at the ED with Mr. Hayes. Jeff said he would give report to a nurse so the ambulance could get back into service. Jeff approached the first person in white that he saw and began to give a quick report on Mr. Hayes. The woman told Jeff that she was not the person to talk to, that he should try the nurse in Room 23.

1. Give at least three reasons why the woman would not accept the report from Jeff.

2. Suggest two ways in which Jeff could have discovered the reasons for the woman to direct him elsewhere.

Critical Thinking 2: Read the scenario and then answer the question.

Jeff had found the correct nurse to give report to but felt that she was not listening to him.

1. Suggest at least two ways in which Jeff could assure himself that the nurse was listening to the report.

Critical Thinking 3: Read the scenario and then answer the questions.

While Jeff was giving the report, the nurse indicated that she would prefer for the patient to answer the questions.

1. Suggest two reasons that the nurse would want to obtain information from the patient directly.

2. List those pieces of information that should have been provided by the EMT to the nurse.

CHAPTER 20
Record

An EMT, as a part of the medical team, is held to the same documentation standards as any other health care provider.

True or False: Read each statement and decide if it is true or false. Place T or F on the line before each statement.

1. ____ The chief complaint is the basis for care.
2. ____ Continuous quality improvement is an ongoing process.
3. ____ Persons who are required by law to report certain situations are mandated reporters.
4. ____ The minimum data set describes what happened to create an injury.
5. ____ The patient care report is a hospital-based form.
6. ____ The patient will sign a special incident report if he refuses care or transport.
7. ____ The agency medical director may review a sentinel PCR.
8. ____ A triage tag is used by the triage nurse to make room assignments.

Fill in the Blank: Complete each sentence using the Key Terms in Chapter 21 of the textbook.

1. Written testimony is made on a(n)______________________________.
2. Information obtained by direct observation or measurement is ______________________________ in nature.
3. The "P" in SOAP stands for ______________________________.
4. A(n) ____________________________ observation is something that the EMT cannot directly see or measure.
5. A(n) ____________________________ observation is something that can be measured.
6. The chief complaint would be an example of ____________________________ information.
7. "The patient fell from the ladder" is an example of the ________________________ ________________ ________________.
8. The document that an EMT would use to describe a stretcher malfunction is the ____________________________ ______________________ ____________________________.

Listing: List four functions of the PCR.

1.
2.
3.
4.

Short Answer: Read each question. Think about the information presented in your text, and then answer each question with one or two sentences.

1. Describe the differences between an open format PCR and a closed format PCR.

2. When is a closed format especially useful?

3. When is an open format useful?

Critical Thinking: Read the following scenario and then document the patient encounter using both SOAP and CHEATED.

XYZ Ambulance Service was sent to the scene of a car that had collided into a tree. Witnesses reported that the car did not try to stop. There were no skid marks noted on the road. The speed limit in the area was 40 mph. The only occupant of the car was the driver, Mr. Kardis. The first responders stated that they removed his seat belt when beginning their assessment. Mr. Kardis complained that it hurt to breathe. He said that his cell phone rang, and when he went to answer it, he became distracted. The EMTs noted that the car was stable, there were no overhanging branches, and the windshield was intact. Mr. Kardis denied losing consciousness. He was speaking clearly, but only at two to three words per breath. His face was drawn tight and he grimaced each time he took a breath. The steering wheel was intact, but the air bag had deployed. Mr. Kardis was breathing 26 times per minute. His pulse rate was 100, and the first responders reported a blood pressure of 116/76. There was no evidence of any broken bones or obvious bleeding. Lung sounds were clear, although it hurt when the stethoscope was placed on the right side of the ribs. Mr. Kardis was started on 15 lpm of oxygen by NRB mask. His C-spine was protected. Collar was applied and a short spine device was used to remove him to a long spine board. He had good extremity pulses and could feel and move all extremities before and after the move. He told the EMTs that he was allergic to penicillin, took a pill for his high blood pressure, and had a hernia operation three years ago. He had just finished lunch and was on his way back to work when the accident occurred.

CHAPTER 21
Head Injuries

Approximately half of the trauma deaths in the United States are due to head injuries. Recognition of the signs and symptoms of a serious head injury is a necessary skill for an EMT. It is crucial that the EMT be familiar with the concepts of managing a patient with a head injury.

Matching: Match the word or term with its definition.

1. _____ basilar skull fracture	a.	a way to quantify level of consciousness
2. _____ Cushing's reflex	b.	bony prominence behind the ear
3. _____ Cushing's triad	c.	a collection of blood
4. _____ Glasgow Coma Scale	d.	blood between the brain and the dura mater
5. _____ intracranial pressure	e.	seizing after head trauma
6. _____ mastoid process	f.	pressure within the skull
7. _____ subdural hematoma	g.	break at the base of skull behind the face
8. _____ epidural hematoma	h.	hypertension/bradycardia after a head injury
9. _____ post-traumatic seizure	i.	blood between the skull and the dura mater
10. _____ hematoma	j.	increased blood pressure, slow heart rate, and altered respiratory patterns after a serious head injury

Identification: Name the sign that is described by each of the following.

1. ____________________ Bruising over the mastoid process after a head injury
2. ____________________ CSF leaking from the ear
3. ____________________ Bruising around both eyes after a head injury
4. ____________________ CSF leaking from the nose
5. ____________________ Increased BP, decreased pulse, and irregular respirations after a head injury

True or False: Read each statement and decide if it is true or false. Place T or F on the line before each statement.

1. _____ Examination of a fontanel is an important assessment skill in both adults and children.
2. _____ The EMT should be able to differentiate a basilar skull fracture from an open one.
3. _____ In an open skull fracture, cover the exposed brain with a saline-soaked dressing.
4. _____ Stabilize an object that has penetrated the skull.
5. _____ The elderly are at increased risk of developing a subdural hematoma after minor trauma.
6. _____ If changes in level of consciousness occur more than 24 hours after the injury, the patient has suffered an epidural hematoma.
7. _____ Bleeding inside the skull can occur in the absence of trauma.
8. _____ The EMT should suspect spinal injury with head trauma.
9. _____ Persistent vomiting is associated with serious head injury.
10. _____ A patient can receive a total of zero (0) on the Glasgow Coma Scale.

Calculation: Calculate the Glasgow Coma Score for each of the following.

1. When called to, patient opens eyes, mumbles sounds, and moves hand away when pinched
2. The patient watches what the EMTs are doing, asks questions about care, and extends arm when told the EMT will take a blood pressure
3. Patient's eyes are closed, makes no sounds, and extends arms and legs stiffly when pinched
4. The patient makes no movement or sounds
5. Patient looks at EMT when spoken to, doesn't know where she is, keeps asking about incident, and pushes the EMT's hand away when pinched

Sorting: Place an X in front of each intervention appropriate to a significantly head-injured patient.

_____ ventilate at up to 20 breaths per minute in the adult patient

_____ elevate the head of the stretcher or board

_____ stop CSF flow

_____ control bleeding

_____ determine exact diagnosis

_____ withhold oxygen

_____ provide rapid transport

_____ avoid helicopter transport due to pressure changes

_____ calculate GCS

Fill in the Blank: Complete the following sentences.

The most important thing an EMT can do to improve the outcome of a head-injured patient is to adequately assess and manage the ____________________, ____________________, and ____________________ status. The brain needs adequate perfusion with well-____________________ blood. After ensuring an adequate airway, assess the effectiveness of the patient's own ____________________. Next, turn attention to the ____________________ status.

For the patient who has suffered a significant injury, the EMT should then move on to a ____________________ ____________________ ____________________. For a high-priority patient, this will be done during transport. During both assessments completed up to this time, the ____________________ of ____________________, or patient responsiveness, will be observed. This can be quantified on the ____________________ ____________________ scale. A ____________________ or pattern that may be seen in repeated vital signs is an increased BP, decreased pulse rate, and changed respiratory pattern. This combination is called ____________________ ____________________.

As with all high priority patients, be sure the patient is receiving high-____________________ ____________________. Ongoing assessments should be completed every 5 minutes.

Short Answer: Read each question. Think about the information presented in your text, and then answer each question with one or two sentences.

1. Why is hypotension so dangerous for a patient with a head injury?

2. What causes the fontanels to bulge?

Critical Thinking 1: Read the following scenario and then answer the questions.

Janice and Brad were assigned to standby at the motorcross rally. They were enjoying the sport when the radio crackled. There was an accident on the first hill. A 12-year-old named Billy was lying on the ground, not moving. Spectators reported that he had missed a jump and struck a tree head first. His helmet, which was nearby, was cracked.

1. Based on the report, what injuries should the EMTs suspect?
2. What interventions must be provided for Billy during the initial assessment?
3. What two methods should the EMTs use to document mental status?
4. List two methods the EMTs can use to reduce brain swelling.

Critical Thinking 2: Read the following scenario and then answer the questions.

Carolyn's mother was upset as she spoke to the EMTs. She and Carolyn were shopping at the mall when Carolyn suddenly collapsed, striking her head hard on the floor. She appeared to have had a seizure. Mall security reported that Carolyn was unresponsive when they first arrived, then awoke briefly and talked with them, complaining of a headache. Now she was unresponsive again.

1. What initial management must be provided for Carolyn?
2. List eight signs of increasing intracranial pressure.
3. What treatment do you expect will occur at the hospital?

CHAPTER 22
Spine Injuries

The immediate care provided to the patient with a spinal injury is critical to prevent further damage from occurring. An EMT is often the primary prehospital caregiver for patients who have sustained spine injuries. It is important that the EMT knows how to recognize that a spinal injury may exist and how to properly care for such a patient.

Word Scramble: Unscramble the following words using the Key Terms in Chapter 22 of the textbook.

1. Inability to move — ssaalypri ________________
2. Cannot move lower extremities — geapipaarl ________________
3. Abnormal sensation — reetasisaph ________________
4. Cannot move four extremities — idregquiplaa ________________
5. Caused by nerve interruption — spaimipr ________________

Identification: Complete the following anatomy review.

________________ Bones of the spinal column

________________ First seven bones of column compose the ___ spine

________________ Portion of the spine behind the chest

________________ Part of spine considered low back

________________ Coverings over cord and brain

Fill in the Blank: Complete the following sentences.

The first clue the EMT has as to the possibility of a spinal injury is the __________ of __________. Knowing the stacked nature of the vertebrae will enable the EMT to imagine the injuries. In a motor vehicle collision, the most common injury type is __________ of the neck. Falls can result in __________ bones that intrude into the cord, or __________ fractures that actually crush the vertebrae. The phenomenon, known as __________ __________, can cause trauma along the spinal column, especially in the lumbar region. Firearms can lead to spinal injuries due to the uncertainty of the __________ of __________ of the bullet. Sports injuries may also cause spinal injury.

True or False: Read each statement and decide if it is true or false. Place T or F on the line before each statement.

1. _____ All spinal injuries will result in nerve deficit.
2. _____ The first clue to a spinal injury is the MOI.
3. _____ Suspicion of spinal injury should be much higher in the elderly.
4. _____ Patients with gunshot injuries to neck or torso should be treated as if they have a spinal cord injury.
5. _____ Alcohol use increases the sensations associated with spinal injury.
6. _____ The inability to move is called paresthesia.
7. _____ Neurogenic shock is characterized by a slow heart rate and warm skin.
8. _____ The first priority of care in a suspected spinal cord injury is to protect the cord.
9. _____ A cervical spine immobilization device is a definitive method of spinal protection.
10. _____ Rapid extrication is for all persons with suspected spinal cord injury.

Short Answer: Read each question. Think about the information presented in your text, and then answer each question with one or two sentences.

1. Explain how it is possible for a patient with a broken vertebra to walk around immediately after an incident.

2. A patient tells you that he has broken his tailbone. Is this possible? Why or why not? Would this result in a spinal cord deficit?

3. Why would a spinal injury in the neck cause greater management difficulties for the EMT than an identical injury located in the lumbar area?

4. Why does a patient with neurogenic shock present differently than one with hypovolemic shock?

5. How would the suspicion of a spinal cord injury alter airway management?

Critical Thinking: Read each of the scenarios and decide how to manage the patient's spine.

1. A 45-year-old man was involved in a low-speed, rear-end collision. He is complaining of neck and shoulder pain. He was wearing both a lap and shoulder harness, he had full movement and sensation of lower extremities, and there was minimal damage to either car.

2. An unrestrained female was involved in a head-on collision into a tree. There were no skid marks, the posted speed limit was 40 mph, and she had difficulty breathing.

3. An 18-year-old male was walking around his damaged Jeep. The vehicle rolled twice on highway, ending up in a ditch. The driver couldn't remember if he was wearing a seat belt. He denies complaints.

Chapter 22 Skill Sheet

Student Name ______________________________ Date ________________

Skill 22-1: Application of the Cervical Spine Immobilization Device

Equipment Needed:

1. Assortment of cervical immobilization devices (collars)
2. Personal protective equipment

Yes: ❑ Reteach: ❑ Return: ❑ Instructor initials: ________

Step 1: Move the patient's head into neutral alignment. If the patient complains of pain, or resistance is felt, then the patient's neck should be splinted in position.

Yes: ❑ Reteach: ❑ Return: ❑ Instructor initials: ________

Step 2: Maintain continuous manual stabilization of the patient's head throughout the procedure.

Yes: ❑ Reteach: ❑ Return: ❑ Instructor initials: ________

Step 3: A second EMT checks for distal pulses, movement, and sensation.

Yes: ❑ Reteach: ❑ Return: ❑ Instructor initials: ________

Step 4: The second EMT measures the patient's neck for a cervical collar, according to manufacturer recommendations.

Yes: ❑ Reteach: ❑ Return: ❑ Instructor initials: ________

Step 5: The second EMT slides the posterior portion of the collar in the void behind the neck.

Yes: ❑ Reteach: ❑ Return: ❑ Instructor initials: ________

Step 6: Cupping the chin piece in one hand, the second EMT slides the anterior portion of the collar up the chest until it captures the chin.

Yes: ❑ Reteach: ❑ Return: ❑ Instructor initials: ________

(continues)

Chapter 22 Skill Sheet

Skill 22-1: *Continued*

Step 7: With collar in place, the second EMT securely fastens the Velcro.

Yes: ❑ Reteach: ❑ Return: ❑ Instructor initials: ________

Step 8: Checking for a proper collar fit, the second EMT mentally draws a line from the opening of the ear to the middle of the shoulder, and from the opening of the ear to the eyes. There should be a 90-degree angle imagined.

Yes: ❑ Reteach: ❑ Return: ❑ Instructor initials: ________

Step 9: The second EMT rechecks for distal pulses, sensation, and movement.

Yes: ❑ Reteach: ❑ Return: ❑ Instructor initials: ________

Step 10: Continuous manual stabilization must be maintained, despite the presence of the cervical immobilization device.

Yes: ❑ Reteach: ❑ Return: ❑ Instructor initials: ________

Chapter 22 Skill Sheet

Student Name ______________________________ Date ________________

Skill 22-2: Application of the Short Immobilization Device

Equipment Needed:

1. Assortment of cervical spine immobilization devices
2. Short immobilization device
3. Personal protective equipment

Yes: ❑ Reteach: ❑ Return: ❑ Instructor initials: ________

Step 1: First, an EMT manually stabilizes the spine. A second EMT then applies a properly sized cervical spine immobilization device. Once the collar is secure, the second EMT checks distal pulses, movement, and sensation.

Yes: ❑ Reteach: ❑ Return: ❑ Instructor initials: ________

Step 2: While a trained assistant maintains continuous manual stabilization throughout the procedure, the EMT places his arms along the anterior and posterior thorax. The patient may now be moved forward as a unit, keeping the spine in line.

Yes: ❑ Reteach: ❑ Return: ❑ Instructor initials: ________

Step 3: The device is then positioned behind the patient cautiously; the patient is leaned back against the device.

Yes: ❑ Reteach: ❑ Return: ❑ Instructor initials: ________

Step 4: Next, the patient's torso, including the legs, is secured to the device.

Yes: ❑ Reteach: ❑ Return: ❑ Instructor initials: ________

Step 5: Finally, the patient's head is secured to the device. The EMT pads the void behind the head as needed.

Yes: ❑ Reteach: ❑ Return: ❑ Instructor initials: ________

Step 6: The EMT then reassesses distal pulses, movement, and sensory function of the patient before transferring the patient to the backboard.

Yes: ❑ Reteach: ❑ Return: ❑ Instructor initials: ________

Chapter 22 Skill Sheet

Student Name ______________________________ Date ________________

Skill 22-3: Rapid Extrication

Equipment Needed:

1. Assortment of cervical spine immobilization devices
2. Long spine board
3. Turnout gear
4. Personal protective equipment

Yes: ❑ Reteach: ❑ Return: ❑ Instructor initials: ________

Step 1: The EMT first checks distal pulses, movement, and sensation. Then the EMT moves the head to a neutral position and has another EMT apply a properly sized cervical collar.

Yes: ❑ Reteach: ❑ Return: ❑ Instructor initials: ________

Step 2: With an EMT on each side of the patient, the patient is gently lifted a couple of inches, so that a long spine board may be inserted under the patient's buttocks.

Yes: ❑ Reteach: ❑ Return: ❑ Instructor initials: ________

Step 3: While an EMT continues to maintain manual stabilization of the spine, one EMT grasps the patient under the arms while another grasps the patient at the hips. Then, on command, the EMTs rotate the patient to side about 45 degrees. At this point, the EMTs may need to switch places if the car's B post becomes an obstruction. After two or three small turns to rotate the patient, the patient should be parallel to the long spine board.

Yes: ❑ Reteach: ❑ Return: ❑ Instructor initials: ________

Step 4: Once the patient is parallel to the long spine board, the patient is lowered, as a stiff unit, to the long spine board while the EMTs maintain in-line stabilization.

Yes: ❑ Reteach: ❑ Return: ❑ Instructor initials: ________

Step 5: Once the patient is on the long spine board, first the body, and then the head, should be fastened securely. The EMT should recheck the patient's distal pulses, movement, and sensation.

Yes: ❑ Reteach: ❑ Return: ❑ Instructor initials: ________

Chapter 22 Skill Sheet

Student Name ______________________ Date ____________

Skill 22-4: Long Axis Drag

Equipment Needed:

Appropriate PPE

Yes: ❑ Reteach: ❑ Return: ❑ Instructor initials: ________

Step 1: First, the EMT determines that the patient needs immediate extrication for some reason; for example, if the patient is in cardiac arrest.

Yes: ❑ Reteach: ❑ Return: ❑ Instructor initials: ________

Step 2: Opening the closest door and entering the passenger compartment, the EMT disentangles any extremities from pedals and other obstructions.

Yes: ❑ Reteach: ❑ Return: ❑ Instructor initials: ________

Step 3: Then the EMT reaches behind the patient's back and under both of the patient's arms to grab the patient's wrists.

Yes: ❑ Reteach: ❑ Return: ❑ Instructor initials: ________

Step 4: The EMT then rotates the patient, as a unit, and places the patient into a semi-inclined position.

Yes: ❑ Reteach: ❑ Return: ❑ Instructor initials: ________

Step 5: The EMT then drags the patient out of the motor vehicle with the patient's head resting on the EMT's forearms.

Yes: ❑ Reteach: ❑ Return: ❑ Instructor initials: ________

Step 6: By dropping to his knees, the EMT can lower the patient and crawl backward with the patient, while performing a long axis drag.

Yes: ❑ Reteach: ❑ Return: ❑ Instructor initials: ________

Chapter 22 Skill Sheet

Student Name ______________________________ Date ________________

Skill 22-5: Modified Logroll of the Supine Patient

Equipment Needed:

1. Selection of cervical collars
2. Long spine board
3. Strapping system
4. Head immobilization system

Yes: ❑ Reteach: ❑ Return: ❑ Instructor initials: ________

Step 1: An EMT checks distal pulses, movement, and sensation of all four extremities, while another EMT maintains manual stabilization.

Yes: ❑ Reteach: ❑ Return: ❑ Instructor initials: ________

Step 2: While one EMT holds manual stabilization, two more EMTs take positions at the patient's shoulders and pelvis, reaching across the patient and grasping the patient's shoulders and pelvis, respectively.

Yes: ❑ Reteach: ❑ Return: ❑ Instructor initials: ________

Step 3: On command, the three EMTs roll the patient on her side. The patient's arms should be at her side.

Yes: ❑ Reteach: ❑ Return: ❑ Instructor initials: ________

Step 4: One EMT pulls the long spine board under the patient. The long spine board should end at the back of the patient's knees.

Yes: ❑ Reteach: ❑ Return: ❑ Instructor initials: ________

Step 5: On command, the patient is rolled back onto the long spine board, and the patient is pulled up to the center of the board, using a long axis drag.

Yes: ❑ Reteach: ❑ Return: ❑ Instructor initials: ________

Step 6: Once the patient is centered on the long spine board, the EMT secures the patient to the long spine board and reassesses distal pulses, movement, and sensation.

Yes: ❑ Reteach: ❑ Return: ❑ Instructor initials: ________

Chapter 22 Skill Sheet

Student Name ______________________________ Date ________________

Skill 22-6: Four-Person Lift

Equipment Needed:

1. Assortment of cervical collars
2. Long spine board
3. Strapping system
4. Head immobilization system

Yes: ❑ Reteach: ❑ Return: ❑ Instructor initials: ________

Step 1: The first EMT kneels at the patient's head and immediately obtains manual stabilization. The second EMT checks the patient's distal pulses, movement, and sensation, and applies a cervical collar.

Yes: ❑ Reteach: ❑ Return: ❑ Instructor initials: ________

Step 2: The second EMT then straddles the patient and drops one knee to the ground. Placing his hands under the patient's arms, he grasps the shoulder girdle.

Yes: ❑ Reteach: ❑ Return: ❑ Instructor initials: ________

Step 3: A third EMT straddles the patient at the hips, and drops his opposite knee to the ground. He then grasps the patient around the hips.

Yes: ❑ Reteach: ❑ Return: ❑ Instructor initials: ________

Step 4: On command, three EMTs gently and evenly lift the patient about two inches, while a fourth EMT slides the long spine board under the patient.

Yes: ❑ Reteach: ❑ Return: ❑ Instructor initials: ________

Step 5: Once the patient is properly positioned, the EMTs proceed to immobilize the torso, and then the head, of the patient. Then the EMT rechecks distal pulses, movement, and sensation.

Yes: ❑ Reteach: ❑ Return: ❑ Instructor initials: ________

Chapter 22 Skill Sheet

Student Name ______________________ Date ____________

Skill 22-7: Long Spine Board Immobilization of the Standing Patient

Equipment Needed:

1. Assortment of cervical collars
2. Long spine board
3. Strapping system
4. Head immobilization system

Yes: ❑ Reteach: ❑ Return: ❑ Instructor initials: ________

Step 1: The EMT approaches the patient from the front and takes immediate anterior head stabilization.

Yes: ❑ Reteach: ❑ Return: ❑ Instructor initials: ________

Step 2: Another EMT takes head stabilization from the rear, while the first EMT assesses distal pulses, movement, and sensation.

Yes: ❑ Reteach: ❑ Return: ❑ Instructor initials: ________

Step 3: An appropriately sized cervical collar is applied to the patient.

Yes: ❑ Reteach: ❑ Return: ❑ Instructor initials: ________

Step 4: Another EMT places the long spine board upright behind the patient and between the arms of the EMT holding stabilization.

Yes: ❑ Reteach: ❑ Return: ❑ Instructor initials: ________

Step 5: One EMT then stands on either side of the patient, holds the board under the patient's arms, and stabilizes the bottom of the board with a foot.

Yes: ❑ Reteach: ❑ Return: ❑ Instructor initials: ________

Step 6: Slowly, the board and the patient are lowered to the ground, while the EMT at the head stabilizes the head and neck. The EMT then immobilizes the patient and rechecks distal pulses, movement, and sensation.

Yes: ❑ Reteach: ❑ Return: ❑ Instructor initials: ________

Chapter 22 Skill Sheet

Student Name ______________________________ Date ________________

Skill 22-8: Helmet Removal

Equipment Needed:

1. Backboard
2. Scissors
3. Assortment of cervical collars

Yes: ❑ Reteach: ❑ Return: ❑ Instructor initials: ________

Step 1: The first EMT manually stabilizes the head in the helmet, while the second EMT assesses distal pulses, movement, and sensation. Any glasses should be removed at this time.

Yes: ❑ Reteach: ❑ Return: ❑ Instructor initials: ________

Step 2: The second EMT then cuts or unfastens the chin strap, slides one hand under the head, stabilizing the head from below, and places his hand on the jaw, stabilizing the head from above.

Yes: ❑ Reteach: ❑ Return: ❑ Instructor initials: ________

Step 3: The first EMT then removes the helmet by spreading the helmet apart gently while moving the helmet from the back of the head.

Yes: ❑ Reteach: ❑ Return: ❑ Instructor initials: ________

Step 4: Once the helmet is completely removed, the first EMT assumes manual stabilization of the head. It may be necessary to pad under the head.

Yes: ❑ Reteach: ❑ Return: ❑ Instructor initials: ________

Step 5: A cervical collar is then fitted to the patient.

Yes: ❑ Reteach: ❑ Return: ❑ Instructor initials: ________

Step 6: With the collar in place, and the head in a neutral position, the EMT rechecks distal pulses, movement, and sensation.

Yes: ❑ Reteach: ❑ Return: ❑ Instructor initials: ________

(continues)

NREMT Skill Sheet

Spinal Immobilization: Seated Patient

Start Time: ____________________

Stop Time: ____________________ **Date:** ____________________

Candidate's Name: ____________________

Evaluator's Name: ____________________

	Points Possible	Points Awarded
Takes, or verbalizes, body substance isolation precautions	1	
Directs assistant to place maintain head in the neutral in-line position	1	
Directs assistant to maintain manual immobilization of the head	1	
Reassesses motor, sensory and circulatory function in each extremity	1	
Applies appropriately sized extrication collar	1	
Positions the immobilization device behind the patient	1	
Secures the device to the patient's torso	1	
Evaluates torso fixation and adjusts as necessary	1	
Evaluates and pads behind the patient's head as necessary	1	
Secures the patient's head to the device	1	
Verbalizes moving the patient to a long board	1	
Reassesses motor, sensory and circulatory function in each extremity	1	
Total:	12	

Critical Criteria

_______ Did not immediately direct, or take, manual immobilization of the head

_______ Released, or ordered release of, manual immobilization before it was maintained mechanically

_______ Patient manipulated, or moved excessively, causing potential spinal compromise

_______ Device moved excessively up, down, left or right on the patient's torso

_______ Head immobilization allows for excessive movement

_______ Torso fixation inhibits chest rise, resulting in respiratory compromise

_______ Upon completion of immobilization, head is not in the neutral position

_______ Did not assess motor, sensory and circulatory function in each extremity after voicing immobilization to the long board

_______ Immobilized head to the board before securing the torso

NREMT Skill Sheet

Spinal Immobilization: Supine Patient

Start Time: ______________________

Stop Time: ______________________ **Date:** ______________

Candidate's Name: ______________________________

Evaluator's Name: ______________________________

	Points Possible	Points Awarded
Takes, or verbalizes, body substance isolation precautions	1	
Directs assistant to place/maintain head in the neutral in-line position	1	
Directs assistant to maintain manual immobilization of the head	1	
Reassesses motor, sensory and circulatory function in each extremity	1	
Applies appropriately sized extrication collar	1	
Positions the immobilization device appropriately	1	
Directs movement of the patient onto the device without compromising the integrity of the spine	1	
Applies padding to voids between the torso and the board as necessary	1	
Immobilizes the patient's torso to the device	1	
Evaluates and pads behind the patient's head as necessary	1	
Immobilizes the patient's head to the device	1	
Secures the patient's legs to the device	1	
Secures the patient's arms to the device	1	
Reassesses motor, sensory and circulatory function in each extremity	1	
Total:	14	

Critical Criteria

_______ Did not immediately direct, or take, manual immobilization of the head

_______ Released, or ordered release of, manual immobilization before it was maintained mechanically

_______ Patient manipulated, or moved excessively, causing potential spinal compromise

_______ Patient moves excessively up, down, left or right on the patient's torso

_______ Head immobilization allows for excessive movement

_______ Upon completion of immobilization, head is not in the neutral position

_______ Did not assess motor, sensory and circulatory function in each extremity after immobilization to the device

_______ Immobilized head to the board before securing the torso

CHAPTER 23
Chest and Abdominal Injuries

Over one-half of all serious trauma patients have chest or abdominal injuries. Prehospital care provided by EMTs has a positive impact on the survival of these patients.

Missing Letters: Complete the puzzle using the Key Terms in Chapter 23 of the textbook.

cardiac **c** _ _ _ _ _ _ _ _ _

h _ _ _ _ _ _ _ _ _

e _ _ _ _ _ _ _ _ _ _ _

sucking _ _ _ **s** _ wound

t _ _ _ _ _ _ _ _

and

_ _ _ _ _ _ _ _ _ **a** _

_ **b** _ _ _ _ _

_ _ _ _ **d** _ _ _ _ _ _ motion

_ _ _ _ **o** _ _ _ _ contusion

subcutaneous _ **m** _ _ _ _ _ _ _

_ _ _ **i** _ segment

_ _ **n** _ _ _ _ _ _ _ _ m _ _ _ _ _ _ _

_ _ _ _ _ _ _ **a** _

_ _ _ _ _ _ _ **l** deviation

Identification: For each of the following signs or symptoms, state whether it is evidence of a simple pneumothorax (**S**), a tension pneumothorax (**T**), or both (**B**).

1. _____ Subcutaneous emphysema
2. _____ Tachycardia
3. _____ Tachypnea
4. _____ Difficulty breathing
5. _____ Diminished breath sounds
6. _____ Jugular venous distension
7. _____ Loss of radial pulses
8. _____ Decreased lung compliance
9. _____ Hypotension
10. _____ Tracheal deviation

Labeling: Label the following organs on the diagram below: heart, lungs, trachea, diaphragm, stomach, liver, small intestines, and bladder.

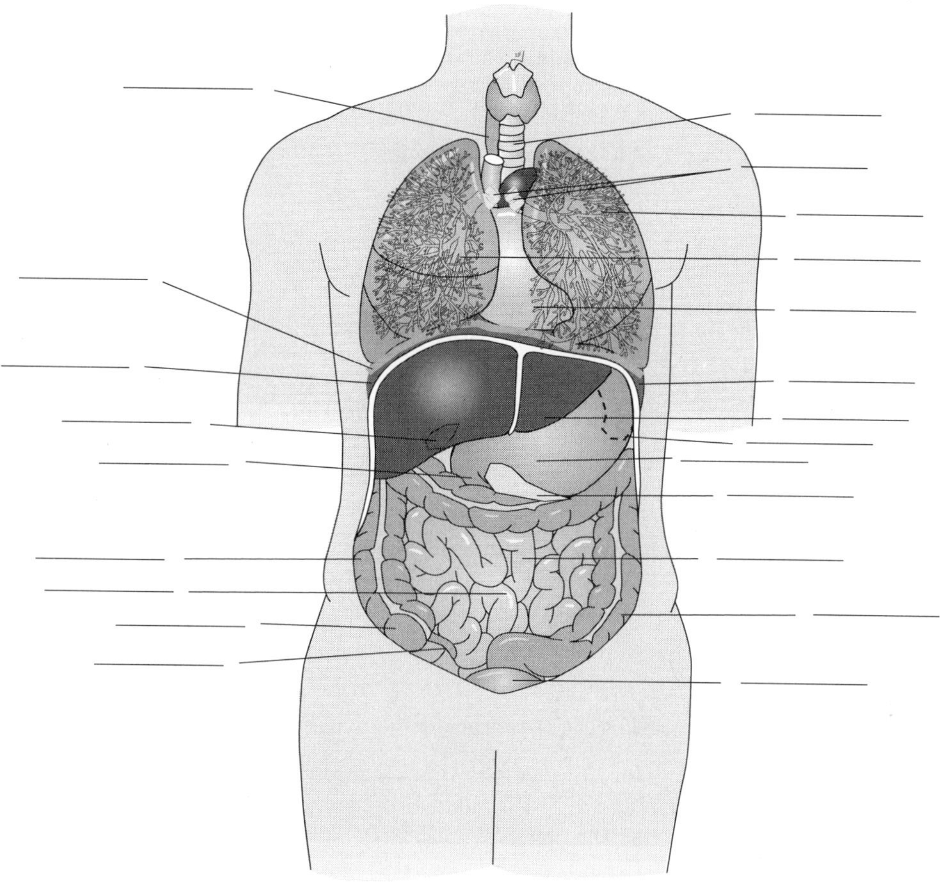

Completion: Complete the missing word or words in each sentence.

1. The most common cause of serious chest injuries is ____________________ trauma.
2. Immediate results of penetrating trauma to the chest are impaired breathing and significant ____________________.
3. The most common signs and symptoms seen in patients with chest injuries are ____________________ and difficulty ____________________.
4. Use the mnemonic ____________________ to help look for injuries.
5. The sign best described as feeling like Rice Krispies is____________________.
6. Management of chest injuries centers on ensuring adequate ventilation, ____________________, and ____________________.
7. Accumulation of blood in the pleural space is called ____________________.
8. The EMT should cover any open wounds to the chest with a(n) ____________________ ____________________.
9. Tape any occlusive dressings on ____________________ sides.
10. Transport the patient with a chest injury on the ____________________ side.

True or False: Read each statement and decide if it is true or false. Place a T or F on the line before each statement.

1. _____ A backup of blood from the heart can cause distended neck veins.
2. _____ A good method of splinting a fractured rib is to let the patient self-splint.
3. _____ Distended neck veins, petechiae, and altered mental status are signs of aortic rupture.

4. _____ Blunt trauma to the abdomen will cause eviscerations.
5. _____ Lower rib injuries may indicate underlying damage to the bladder.
6. _____ Extrusion of the intestines outside the abdominal wall is called abdominal asphyxiation.
7. _____ The EMT must try to replace intestines that protrude through a wound.
8. _____ Moist, sterile dressings should be used to cover eviscerations.
9. _____ A major complication of pelvic fracture is hemorrhaging.
10. _____ Seat belts worn properly can leave contusions.

Short Answer: Read each question. Think about the information presented in your text, and then answer each question with one or two sentences.

1. Why is it unimportant for the EMT to diagnose the actual abdominal injury in the field?

2. Why is it important to cover exposed abdominal organs with moist, sterile dressings and a covering?

Critical Thinking: Read the following scenario and then answer the questions.

Eve and James were dispatched to a local dance hall for "injuries following a fight, shots fired." The sheriff's patrol apprehended the shooter and secured the weapon. At the dance hall, the EMTs found a young man sitting in a chair, clutching his chest. He was screaming at the sheriff that they had better "put that guy away for life."

1. What do the EMTs know about their patient already?

The EMTs talked to the man while removing his shirt. He stated he was sitting in that chair when "this guy started screaming and waving a gun." Next thing he knew, he had been shot. James said he could visualize a small wound to the right side of the chest, approximately 10 inches below the patient's shoulder. There was a larger exit wound to the back in the same region.

2. What are the likely injuries?

3. How should the EMTs manage this patient?

4. How should he be transported?

During transport, he stated he could not breathe at all.

5. What should the EMTs do now?

CHAPTER 24
Soft Tissue Injuries

Uncontrolled bleeding can lead to shock and even death. Fortunately, most bleeding is easily controlled using some very simple maneuvers.

Missing Letters: Complete the puzzle by using the Key Terms in Chapter 24 of the textbook.

s _ _ _ _ _ _ _

o _ _ _

_ _ _ _ f _ _ _ _

t _ _ _ _ _ _ _ _

t _ _ _ _ _   _ _ _ _ _ _ _ _

_ _ _ _   _ _   _ i _ _ _

s _ _ _ _ _ _

s _ _ _ _ _   _ _ _ _ _ _ _

_ _ u _ _

_ _ _ _ _ _ _ _ e _

_ _ i _ _ _ _ _ _   _ _ _ _ _ _ _ _

_ _ _ _ n _ _ _ _ _   _ _ _ _ _ _ _ _

_ _ _ _ _ _ _ _   _ _ j _ _ _

_ _ _ _ _ u _ _

_ _ _ _ r _ _ _ _ _ _   _ _ _ _

_ _ _ _ _ _ i _ _   _ _ _ _ _ _ _ _

_ _ _ _ e _   _ _ _ _ _ _

_ _ _ _ s _ _ _   _ _ _ _ _ _ _ _

Identification: Read each of the following and then write on the line the name of the bandage or dressing described.

1. ____________________ A triangle folded into a band
2. ____________________ A strip of cloth that holds a dressing in place
3. ____________________ Sterile cotton weave cloth
4. ____________________ A 36" by 42", three-sided piece of cloth
5. ____________________ Any sterile, absorbent cloth
6. ____________________ A circumferential cloth holding a chest dressing
7. ____________________ An added layer that directly pushes on the wound
8. ____________________ A cylinder of cloth continually folding back onto itself
9. ____________________ An impenetrable covering
10. ____________________ A cotton dressing with two tails for tying

11. ____________________ Cloth laid back and forth across tape, then anchored
12. ____________________ A cylinder of cloth used for ease in application
13. ____________________ A cylinder of cloth applied around a limb
14. ____________________ A 9" by 36" multilayered cloth
15. ____________________ A constricting band

Definitions: Write the definitions of the following terms.

1. hemorrhage

2. inflammation

3. necrotic

4. coagulation

5. ecchymosis

6. fasciotomy

True or False: Read each statement and decide if it is true or false. Place T or F on the line before each statement.

1. _____ Bleeding can lead to shock.
2. _____ The first step in controlling bleeding is elevation.
3. _____ A tourniquet is useful for controlling capillary bleeding.
4. _____ The pressure point is located within the wound itself.
5. _____ To adequately compress blood vessels, apply an occlusive dressing.
6. _____ Elevation decreases pressure in the vessels serving the wound area.
7. _____ BSI is necessary when caring for a wound.
8. _____ If blood seeps through the first dressing, take it off and apply a new one.

Sorting: Place each descriptor of bleeding into the correct category.

constant	pulsing
watery	pouring out of wound
seeping	oozing
spurting	bright red
deep red	rivulets

Arterial bleeding	**Venous bleeding**	**Capillary bleeding**

Calculation: Using the rule of nines or the palmer method, calculate the percentage of burn.

1. The entire right leg of an adult
2. The front of both arms, front of the chest, and front of the abdomen of an adult
3. Front and back of both legs and the genitalia of a one-year-old child
4. The bottom of the foot of an adult
5. Back of the chest and lower back of an adult
6. A child's palm
7. Entire head of a child
8. The entire left leg, abdomen, and front of left arm of an adult
9. A 2" by 3" section on the front of an adult's abdomen
10. Front of the neck, face, and half of the top of the head on an adult

Identification: Write the correct classification of burn on the line.

1. ______________________________ Reddened
2. ______________________________ Little damage to living tissue
3. ______________________________ Charred
4. ______________________________ Swollen
5. ______________________________ Destruction of nerve endings
6. ______________________________ Painless
7. ______________________________ Leathery
8. ______________________________ Loss of muscle and fat
9. ______________________________ Blistered
10. ______________________________ Flat but painful

Short Answer: Read each question. Think about the information presented in your text, and then answer each question with one or two sentences.

1. A patient receives a partial thickness burn from hot steam used to sterilize equipment. Why is he at risk for infection?

2. Why is it important to concentrate on finding all injuries, instead of just locating the exit and entrance wounds from a gunshot?

3. An EMT is taught to leave an impaled object in place. What can happen if it is removed?

4. Regarding an impaled object, why is the cheek treated differently?

Critical Thinking 1: Read the following scenario and then answer the questions.

Kim and Christina were dispatched to the local industrial park for a worker injured and bleeding. Upon their arrival, they found Mark, a 24-year-old laborer, sitting on a pallet holding onto his neck. The front of his shirt was dark red. The local police were also on scene. Mark's foreman had been opening boxes, when he hit a metal tie. This caused the razor to slip and he hit Mark with it. Kim and Christina took BSI and began their initial assessment.

1. What are the two major concerns for Mark at this point?

2. What treatments must the EMTs provide for Mark during the initial assessment?

3. Once they provide those treatments, why is Mark at great risk for hypoxia?

Critical Thinking 2: Read the following scenario and then answer the questions.

Genna and Andy were staged around the corner from a domestic fight. The dispatch information was that one adult had been stabbed in the chest with an ice pick. The EMTs discussed the likely injuries to result from such an incident. Genna mentioned that they needed to carefully assess for air moving in and out of the chest wound.

1. What type of wound has occurred if air is moving in and out of the chest through the wound?

2. What problems are present for the patient with this type of injury?

3. What treatments must Genna and Andy provide for the patient if this type of injury is present?

CHAPTER 25
Bony Injuries

Most bone injuries are not life-threatening. Careful attention by the EMT to the assessment and management of bone injuries can reduce suffering, prevent further injury, and ultimately assist the patient to a return to health.

Identification: Refer to Chapter 25 to complete the following exercise. List the important bones in each region of the body.

1. Upper and lower arm

2. Wrist and hand

3. Upper and lower leg

4. Ankle and foot

5. Trunk

Definitions: Write the definitions of the following terms.

1. closed fracture ____________________
2. dislocation ____________________
3. dorsiflexion ____________________
4. footdrop ____________________
5. locked ____________________
6. motor nerves ____________________
7. open fracture ____________________
8. osteoporosis ____________________
9. position of function ____________________
10. range of motion ____________________
11. sciatic nerve ____________________
12. sensory nerve ____________________
13. spontaneous reduction ____________________
14. sprain ____________________
15. traction ____________________

Matching: Match each bone injury to its splinting procedure.

1. _____ clavicle
2. _____ mid-lower arm
3. _____ wrist
4. _____ pelvis
5. _____ mid-upper leg
6. _____ patella
7. _____ ankle

a. flexible splint
b. traction splint
c. MAST/PASG or a wrap technique
d. pillow splint
e. a pair of padded board splints
f. sling and swathe
g. rigid splint

True or False: Read each statement and decide if it is true or false. Place T or F on the line before each statement.

1. _____ Splinting an injury should take place immediately.
2. _____ It is best to manually stabilize a suspected fracture before applying any device.
3. _____ Place straps or cravats directly over the injured site.
4. _____ Control any bleeding before splinting.
5. _____ Evaluate pulses, movement, and sensation proximal to the injury.
6. _____ Check for weight-bearing ability before and after splinting.
7. _____ BSI is necessary when caring for an open fracture.
8. _____ Place padding into the spaces between limb and splint.
9. _____ Reassess the limb after splinting.
10. _____ Attempt to splint in position found.
11. _____ Expose the injured limb before splinting.
12. _____ Do not elevate an injured leg.
13. _____ Immobilize the joints above and below a suspected fracture.
14. _____ In a suspected dislocation, realign the joint if pulses are present.
15. _____ Loss of pulses after splinting may be due to tight bandages.

Fill in the Blank: Complete the following sentences on signs and symptoms of bone injuries by filling in the missing word or words.

Next to most _______________ _______________ lies an artery, a _______________, and a _______________. Surrounding the bone are muscles, _______________, and soft tissues. Covering all of this is skin. If a broken bone end cuts an artery, there will be bleeding into the tissues, causing the area to become _______________, _______________, and _______________. Disruption of an artery can cause loss of _______________ distal to the injury.

If a sensory nerve is injured, the patient may complain of numbness or tingling, called _______________. If the motor nerve has been injured, however, the EMT may see signs of weakness of movement or _______________. If there is no movement of the extremity or _______________, check the opposite extremity. Loss of movement on both sides should alert the EMT to possible _______________ injury.

A grating sensation called _______________ can often be noted when the patient moves an injured extremity. This is caused by bone ends _______________ against each other. It is not necessary for the EMT to elicit this! Sudden pain at the exact location of the injury is called _______________ _______________.

During the general impression, the EMT may notice that the patient is protecting or self-splinting an injury. This is called _______________.

Listing: List the 10 signs or symptoms of a suspected fracture.

1. ______________________________
2. ______________________________
3. ______________________________
4. ______________________________
5. ______________________________
6. ______________________________
7. ______________________________
8. ______________________________
9. ______________________________
10. ______________________________

Reviewing: List the word associated with each letter of the mnemonic for assessing injuries.

1. D ____________________
2. C ____________________
3. A ____________________
4. P ____________________
5. B ____________________
6. T ____________________
7. L ____________________
8. S ____________________

Short Answer: Read each question. Think about the information presented in your text, and then answer each question with one or two sentences.

1. Why must the EMT immobilize the joints above and below a suspected fracture site?

2. Why should the EMT splint a suspected dislocated joint in the position found?

3. Explain why a wilderness EMT may need to realign a dislocation before transporting the patient. Is this the same or different for an EMT functioning in a large city? Why?

Critical Thinking 1: Read the following scenario and then answer the questions.

Dan and Greg were called to the scene of a motorcross bike rally. There they found Michael, a 16-year-old who had injured his arm while fixing a bike. Michael was seated at the first-aid station, holding his left arm close to his body.

1. What do the EMTs know about Michael from this encounter?

Michael had caught his left forearm in a spring-loaded piece of equipment. A fellow biker had released the equipment and assisted Michael to the first-aid station. There was no loss of consciousness or fall with this injury.

2. Describe the trauma assessment that Dan and Greg should follow in managing this situation.

The results of the assessment showed that Michael had a swollen, deformed, and painful left forearm. There was point tenderness at approximately the mid-forearm, and crepitus was noted when Michael tried to shift his arm. Michael could wiggle his fingers, feel touch to his hand, and there was a strong radial pulse felt.

3. Describe the management of this injury, including the splinting procedure.

4. Would Dan and Greg need to treat Michael differently if there was a laceration with bleeding observed over the area of point tenderness? If so, how?

5. How would the management change if there were no radial pulses noted on Michael's left arm?

Critical Thinking 2: Read the following scenario and then answer the questions.

Nora and Chris were called to the local high school for Brent, a center for the varsity basketball team. Brent had been playing hard when he could not bear weight on his right leg, and slumped to the floor in a seated position. He told the coach that it felt like his knee had given way, and that he could not move it. When Nora and Chris arrived, Brent was seated on the bench, splinting his knee, his right leg extended. Initial exam showed no life threats. The detailed trauma exam showed deformity to the right knee with swelling on the lateral aspect, inability to move the right leg, strong pedal pulse, and good sensation. The EMTs splinted the knee in the position found and transported Brent to the ED. They reported that Brent had a dislocated knee.

1. Do you agree or disagree with the assessment of a dislocated knee? If you disagree, what is the likely injury?

2. Do you agree or disagree with the management of Brent's injury? If you disagree, how would you manage the injury?

Chapter 25 Skill Sheet

Student Name ______________________________ Date ______________

Skill 25-1: Application of a Unipolar Traction Splint

Equipment Needed:

1. Scissors
2. Unipolar traction device
3. Personal protective equipment

Yes: ❑ Reteach: ❑ Return: ❑ Instructor initials: ________

Step 1: Apply manual stabilization of the limb, while instructing a trained assistant to grasp the leg and apply manual stabilization of the affected leg.

Yes: ❑ Reteach: ❑ Return: ❑ Instructor initials: ________

Step 2: Check distal pulses, movement, and circulation in the affected leg.

Yes: ❑ Reteach: ❑ Return: ❑ Instructor initials: ________

Step 3: Prepare the traction device, adjusting it to about 3–4 inches past the leg.

Yes: ❑ Reteach: ❑ Return: ❑ Instructor initials: ________

Step 4: Slide the traction splint between the legs, and secure the ischial strap across the thigh.

Yes: ❑ Reteach: ❑ Return: ❑ Instructor initials: ________

Step 5: Apply the ankle hitch to the ankle, and apply traction of the leg.

Yes: ❑ Reteach: ❑ Return: ❑ Instructor initials: ________

Step 6: In the last step, place the straps in place, and recheck distal pulses, movement, and sensation.

Yes: ❑ Reteach: ❑ Return: ❑ Instructor initials: ________

Chapter 25 Skill Sheet

Student Name ______________________________ Date ________________

Skill 25-2: Application of a Bipolar Traction Splint

Equipment Needed:

1. Bipolar traction splint
2. Personal protective equipment
3. Scissors

Yes: ❑ Reteach: ❑ Return: ❑ Instructor initials: ________

Step 1: Apply manual stabilization of the limb, while instructing a trained assistant to grasp the leg and apply manual stabilization of the affected leg.

Yes: ❑ Reteach: ❑ Return: ❑ Instructor initials: ________

Step 2: Check distal pulses, movement, and circulation in the affected leg.

Yes: ❑ Reteach: ❑ Return: ❑ Instructor initials: ________

Step 3: Prepare the traction device, adjusting it beyond the length of the uninjured leg, and move the straps into place.

Yes: ❑ Reteach: ❑ Return: ❑ Instructor initials: ________

Step 4: Apply the ankle hitch to the ankle, and assume traction of the leg.

Yes: ❑ Reteach: ❑ Return: ❑ Instructor initials: ________

Step 5: Slide the traction splint under the legs, and secure the ischial strap across the thigh.

Yes: ❑ Reteach: ❑ Return: ❑ Instructor initials: ________

Step 6: In the last step, apply the ankle hitch to the ratchet and apply mechanical traction. With the straps in place, recheck distal pulses, movement, and sensation.

Yes: ❑ Reteach: ❑ Return: ❑ Instructor initials: ________

(continues)

NREMT Skill Sheet

Immobilization Skills: Long Bone Injury

Start Time: ____________________

Stop Time: ____________________ **Date:** ____________________

Candidate's Name: ____________________

Evaluator's Name: ____________________

	Points Possible	Points Awarded
Takes, or verbalizes, body substance isolation precautions	1	
Directs application of manual stabilization of the injury	1	
Assesses motor, sensory and circulatory function in the injured extremity	1	
Note: The examiner acknowledges "motor, sensory and circulatory functions are present and normal."		
Measures the splint	1	
Applies the splint	1	
Immobilizes the joint above the injury site	1	
Immobilizes the joint below the injury site	1	
Secures the entire injured extremity	1	
Immobilizes the hand/foot in the position of function	1	
Reassesses motor, sensory and circulatory function in the injured extremity	1	
Note: The examiner acknowledges "motor, sensory and circulatory functions are present and normal."		
Total:	10	

Critical Criteria

_______ Grossly moves the injured extremity

_______ Did not immobilize the joint above and the joint below the injury site

_______ Did not reassess motor, sensory and circulatory function in the injured extremity before and after splinting

NREMT Skill Sheet

Immobilization Skills: Joint Injury

Start Time: ____________________

Stop Time: ____________________ **Date:** ____________________

Candidate's Name: ____________________

Evaluator's Name: ____________________

	Points Possible	Points Awarded
Takes, or verbalizes, body substance isolation precautions	1	
Directs application of manual stabilization of the shoulder injury	1	
Assesses motor, sensory and circulatory function in the injured extremity	1	
Note: The examiner acknowledges "motor, sensory and circulatory functions are present and normal."		
Selects the proper splinting material	1	
Immobilizes the site of the injury	1	
Immobilizes the bone above the injured joint	1	
Immobilizes the bone below the injured joint	1	
Reassesses motor, sensory and circulatory function in the injured extremity	1	
Note: The examiner acknowledges "motor, sensory and circulatory functions are present and normal."		
Total:	8	

Critical Criteria

_______ Did not support the joint so that the joint did not bear distal weight

_______ Did not immobilize the above and below the injured site

_______ Did not reassess motor, sensory and circulatory function in the injured extremity before and after splinting

NREMT Skill Sheet

Immobilization Skills: Traction Splinting

Start Time: ______________________

Stop Time: ______________________ **Date:** ______________

Candidate's Name: ______________________________

Evaluator's Name: ______________________________

	Points Possible	Points Awarded
Takes, or verbalizes, body substance isolation precautions	1	
Directs application of manual stabilization of the injured leg	1	
Directs the application of manual traction	1	
Assesses motor, sensory and circulatory function in the injured extremity	1	
Note: The examiner acknowledges "motor, sensory and circulatory function are present and normal."		
Prepares/adjusts splint to the proper length	1	
Positions the splint next to the injured leg	1	
Applies the proximal securing device (e.g. … ischial strap)	1	
Applies the distal securing device (e.g. … ankle hitch)	1	
Applies mechanical traction	1	
Positions/secures the support straps	1	
Re-evaluates the proximal/distal securing devices	1	
Reassesses motor, sensory and circulatory function in the injured extremity	1	
Note: The examiner acknowledges "motor, sensory and circulatory function are present and normal."		
Note: The examiner must ask the candidate how he/she would prepare the patient for transportation.		
Verbalizes securing the torso to the long board to immobilize the hip	1	
Verbalizes securing the splint to the long board to prevent movement of the splint	1	
Total:	14	

Critical Criteria

_______ Loss of traction at any point after it was applied

_______ Did not reassess motor, sensory and circulatory function in the injured extremity before and after splinting

_______ The foot was excessively rotated or extended after splint was applied

_______ Did not secure the ischial strap before taking traction

_______ Final immobilization failed to support the femur or prevent rotation of the injured leg

_______ Secured the leg to the splint before applying mechanical traction

Note: If the Sagar splint or the Kendricks Traction Device is used without elevating the patient's leg, application of manual traction is not necessary. The candidate should be awarded one (1) point as if manual traction were applied.

Note: If the leg is elevated at all, manual traction must be applied before elevating the leg. The ankle hitch may be applied before elevating the leg and used to provide manual traction.

CHAPTER 26 Medication Administration for the EMT

The study of medications and their interactions is called pharmacology. The EMT-B is responsible for basic pharmacology related to commonly encountered medicines.

Identification: Read the definitions. Write the correct word or terms on the line.

1. ____________________ A specific circumstance in which not to give a drug
2. ____________________ Medications that open narrowed airways
3. ____________________ Instructions to guide treatment decisions
4. ____________________ Effects of a medication
5. ____________________ Amount of the medication given
6. ____________________ Last date that the drug is guaranteed to be effective
7. ____________________ Physician input into writing protocols
8. ____________________ An unintended drug effect
9. ____________________ Reason for giving a medication
10. ____________________ Protocols that can be followed without speaking with a physician

Identification: Place a checkmark in front of each word that is a generic name for a drug.

____ ventolin	____ pseudoephedrine	____ acetaminophen
____ ibuprofen	____ sudafed	____ motrin
____ advil	____ albuterol	____ tylenol

True or False: Read each statement and decide if it is true or false. Place T or F on the line before each statement.

1. _____ Give oxygen based on the oxygen saturation reading.
2. _____ For suspected low blood sugar in an awake patient, give instaglucose.
3. _____ Administer activated charcoal to an unconscious poisoned patient.
4. _____ Assist a patient in respiratory distress to use his albuterol inhaler.
5. _____ Assist a hypotensive patient with chest pain to take a nitro tab.
6. _____ Administer a friend's EpiPen to a patient stung by a bee.
7. _____ Assist a child in holding the oxygen mask.
8. _____ Give activated charcoal to a child who ate Tylenol tabs yesterday.

Identification: For each description, write the name of the drug form.

1. ________________ A powder compressed into a shape
2. ________________ A temperature-sensitive, thick fluid that can be administered and absorbed from the mouth
3. ________________ A powder that floats in a liquid and is more palatable
4. ________________ A powder that floats on air and is inhaled into the lungs
5. ________________ Oxygen is the primary medicinal one

Naming: For each description, write the correct route of administration.

1. ______________ Inside the veins of the body
2. ______________ Inside the mouth
3. ______________ Space just under the skin
4. ______________ Into the deep muscle
5. ______________ Creating a mist to be inhaled
6. ______________ Under the tongue

Listing: List the five rights of drug administration.

1. ____
2. ____
3. ____
4. ____
5. ____

Fill in the Blank: Read the following paragraph on documentation and complete the sentences.

The EMT-B must ____________ the patient and include physical and historical information on the patient care record. List the exact _____________ of the drug, the ____________, or how much was given, and the _______________, or the way it was given. Within five minutes of giving the medication, a ____________________ of the patient should be done and findings from this should be included on the patient care record. Be sure to evaluate the signs or symptoms that led to the use of the medication originally.

Completion: Complete the following table.

Drug indications	Contraindications	Actions	Side effects	Dose/route
charcoal				
oral glucose				
oxygen				
albuterol				
nitroglycerin				
epinephrine				

Critical Thinking 1: Read the scenario. Determine which drug the patient should have, give at least one reason for the patient to have that drug, and list the things that must be reassessed after giving the drug.

Rhonda and Geoff were dispatched to the home of an elderly man who was having difficulty breathing. When they arrived, they found him sitting straight upright in a chair. He could only say one word per breath. He admitted that he was afraid to move because he wouldn't be able to get enough air. Physical exam showed wheezing in both lungs, use of accessory muscles for breathing, a respiratory rate of 24 and labored, a pulse of 88 and regular, and a blood pressure of 136/88. The difficulty breathing began that day when the man had been outside working in his garden during a spell of hot, humid weather. His past medical history included asthma, chronic lung disease, and angina. He had his own albuterol inhaler, nitroglycerin tabs, and aspirin but had not taken any because they were upstairs in the medicine chest.

Critical Thinking 2: Read the scenario. Determine which drug the patient should have, give at least one reason for the patient to have that drug, and list the things that must be reassessed after giving the drug.

Joel and Rick had been called for a woman having difficulty breathing. When they arrived, they found her seated in a chair with a very anxious look on her face. She was flushed in appearance with a raised rash on her face, neck, and arms. Her friends reported that they had been outside playing tennis when a ball went out of bounds into the brush. When the patient came from retrieving it, she complained of a stinging sensation on her leg. Soon after, her speech became thick, and she complained of being dizzy. An exam showed extensive wheezing in both lungs. The friends showed Rick the patient's medications, which included an autoinjector of epinephrine, a metered dose inhaler without a drug name on it, and an antismoking patch.

Critical Thinking 3: Read the scenario. Determine which drug the patient should have, give at least one reason for the patient to have that drug, and list the things that must be reassessed after giving the drug.

Sean and Todd went to the home of a middle-aged woman who complained of having difficulty breathing. When they arrived there, they found her holding her chest. She said she could not get enough air in because it felt like an elephant was seated on her chest. Her past medical history included asthma, diabetes, and angina. The physical exam showed an open airway and clear lungs, with vital signs of BP 134/80, pulse 96, and regular and nonlabored respirations of 18. She had not taken any of her medications, which included nitro tabs, an albuterol inhaler, and insulin.

Chapter 26 Skill Sheet

Student Name ________________________________ Date _______________

Skill 26-1: Assistance with a Metered Dose Inhaler

Equipment Needed:

Appropriate prescribed metered dose inhaler

Yes: ❑ Reteach: ❑ Return: ❑ Instructor initials: ________

Step 1: Assess the patient and apply oxygen, as appropriate.

Yes: ❑ Reteach: ❑ Return: ❑ Instructor initials: ________

Step 2: Confirm that the inhaler is the patient's prescribed inhaler, and check the expiration date.

Yes: ❑ Reteach: ❑ Return: ❑ Instructor initials: ________

Step 3: Shake the inhaler vigorously and remove the mouthpiece.

Yes: ❑ Reteach: ❑ Return: ❑ Instructor initials: ________

Step 4: After removing the oxygen mask, ask the patient to exhale, then to inhale slowly and deeply as you depress the inhaler for one puff.

Yes: ❑ Reteach: ❑ Return: ❑ Instructor initials: ________

Step 5: Remove the inhaler from the patient's mouth, reapply oxygen, and instruct the patient to hold his breath for several seconds. Reevaluate the patient and consider whether a second dose of medicine is needed.

Yes: ❑ Reteach: ❑ Return: ❑ Instructor initials: ________

Chapter 26 Skill Sheet

Student Name ______________________________ Date ______________

Skill 26-2: Assistance with an Epinephrine Auto-Injector

Equipment Needed:

1. Oxygen
2. Prescribed epinephrine auto-injector
3. Scissors
4. Sharps container

Yes: ❑ Reteach: ❑ Return: ❑ Instructor initials: ________

Step 1: Assess the patient and apply oxygen, as appropriate.

Yes: ❑ Reteach: ❑ Return: ❑ Instructor initials: ________

Step 2: Confirm that the auto-injector is the patient's prescribed auto-injector and check the expiration date.

Yes: ❑ Reteach: ❑ Return: ❑ Instructor initials: ________

Step 3: Bare the patient's lateral thigh (using scissors to cut away clothing if necessary) and then remove the safety cap on the auto-injector.

Yes: ❑ Reteach: ❑ Return: ❑ Instructor initials: ________

Step 4: Press the auto-injector firmly against the patient's lateral thigh, midway between the knee and the hip, allowing 10 seconds for medication administration.

Yes: ❑ Reteach: ❑ Return: ❑ Instructor initials: ________

Step 5: Remove the auto-injector and properly dispose of it in a sharps container at the patient's side.

Yes: ❑ Reteach: ❑ Return: ❑ Instructor initials: ________

Step 6: Reassess the patient and initiate transport as soon as possible. Arrange for an ALS intercept if possible.

Yes: ❑ Reteach: ❑ Return: ❑ Instructor initials: ________

CHAPTER 27
Shortness of Breath

Difficulty breathing can be caused by many different problems. Each of these problems may result from a different disease, even though they all cause dysfunction of the respiratory system.

Word Scramble: Using the Key Terms in Chapter 27 of the textbook, unscramble the following words.

1. hasmat ____________________
2. oobcarmpsh ____________________
3. eacclrks ____________________
4. pruco ____________________
5. scaysoni ____________________
6. idisfonuf ____________________
7. peadsny ____________________
8. tttiiipegols ____________________
9. corhnhi ____________________
10. ezghwine ____________________

Fill in the Blank: Complete the missing word or words in each sentence.

1. When in distress, a patient will use ____________________ ____________________ of ____________________, located in the chest and neck to help with breathing.
2. ____________________ ____________________ ____________________ ____________________ describes the movement of oxygen and carbon dioxide between the lungs and the blood.
3. The process allowing the exchange of gas in the periphery is ____________________ ____________________.
4. ____________________ ____________________ ____________________ ____________________, or COPD, is a group of diseases characterized by airway obstruction and bronchospasm.
5. Backup of pressure from the left side of the heart causing fluids to leak into the alveoli describes ____________________ ____________________ ____________________.
6. Low levels of oxygen stimulate breathing in a patient on ____________________ ____________________.
7. A blockage in the pulmonary arterial circulation disrupting gas exchange is called a ____________________ ____________________.
8. Gas exchange is called ____________________, while movement of air in and out of the lungs is ____________________.

Sorting: List the characteristics found in children or adults, or both, by placing each in the correct category.

very flexible trachea
floppy large epiglottis
15–30 breaths per minute
easily obstructed by slight swelling
tongue takes up most of mouth
wheezing
12–20 breaths per minute

Pediatric **Adult** **Both**

Matching: Match each word or term with its definition.

1. _____ croup
2. _____ epiglottitis
3. _____ pulmonary embolus
4. _____ CHF
5. _____ COPD
6. _____ asthma
7. _____ dyspnea

a. feeling it is difficult to breathe
b. hyperreactive airway disease
c. viral infection of kids causing barking cough
d. infection of tissues above the larynx
e. airways open, blood flow in lungs impaired
f. chronic disorder of airways
g. fluid-filled alveoli

Short Answer: For each of the diseases, list at least one risk factor.

1. Pulmonary embolus _______________
2. COPD _______________
3. Asthma _______________
4. Croup _______________
5. Epiglottitis _______________

Completion: Complete the following drug card for an albuterol inhaler.

Generic name albuterol
Trade name _______________
Indication _______________
Contraindication _______________
Dose _______________
Route _______________

Labeling: Identify the following structures on the diagram.

Nose _______________
Mouth _______________
Pharynx _______________
Larynx _______________
Trachea _______________
Right lung _______________
Bronchus _______________
Bronchiole _______________
Alveoli _______________

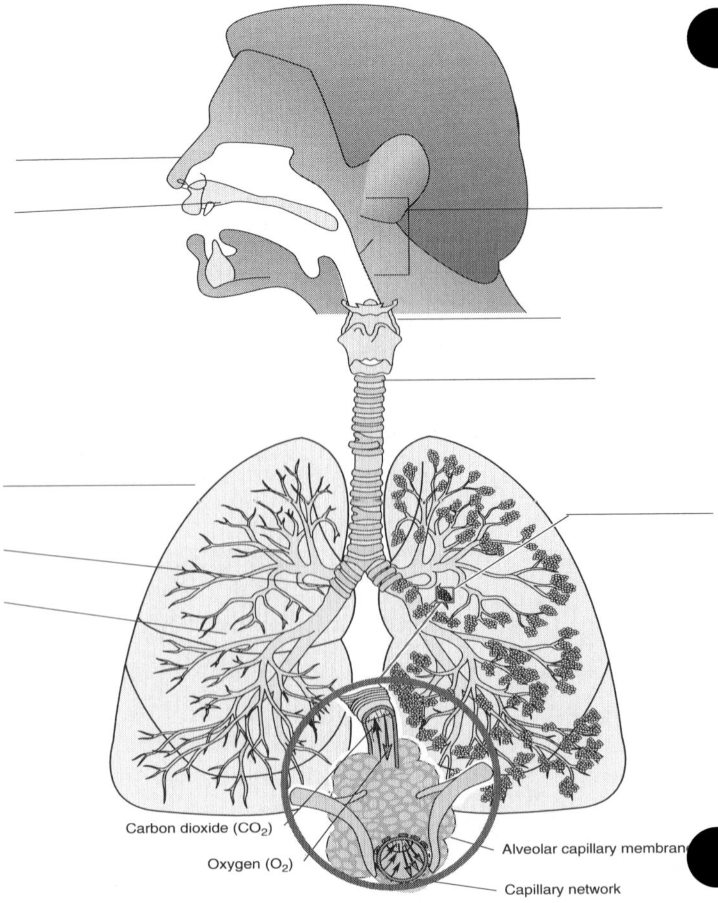

Short Answer: Read each question. Think about the information presented in your text, and then answer each question with one or two sentences.

1. Why does the body eventually switch to hypoxic drive?

2. Explain why the body doesn't switch to hypoxic drive in hypoperfusion.

Critical Thinking 1: Read the following scenario and then answer the questions.

As the weather got colder, Diane and Jim found themselves answering more and more calls for difficulty breathing. This was the one they feared. Dispatch was for a 2-year-old experiencing difficulty in breathing. When they arrived, they found a calm but worried mother holding her 2-year-old daughter, Kara. Kara's wheezing could be heard without a stethoscope. She had a cold that had gotten worse over the course of last evening. Her mother had tried to manage it with prescribed medications and mist from the shower in the bathroom. Kara had continued to get worse, and so 9-1-1 was called.

While Jim asked Kara's mother questions, Diane applied oxygen and continued her assessment. Kara had a history of asthma and normally took Ventolin syrup; she could be given a nebulizer treatment of Ventolin by her mother as well. She was otherwise a healthy, happy little girl. When Kara's asthma was diagnosed, her family had given their kitten to the neighbors and Kara had not had an attack in over six months.

Diane and Jim moved Kara and her mother to the ambulance and strapped them in for safety. Diane began an ongoing assessment and determined that Kara's respiratory rate had dropped from 32 breaths per minute to 12 per minute, and that the wheezing was very difficult to hear. Kara was also now difficult to awaken.

1. Why was Kara wheezing?

2. Why was Diane unable to hear wheezing when she continued her assessment?

3. What treatment must Diane begin now for Kara?

Critical Thinking 2: Read the following scenario and then answer the questions.

Christina was a good EMT. When she heard her son Adam coughing during the night, she recognized the characteristic bark of croup. She also knew that she would need help. Adam had a cold for several days and was slightly feverish before he went to bed the previous evening. Now he was sounding like a seal and seemed to have difficulty catching his breath.

Christina took him into the bathroom and turned on the shower while she called 9-1-1.

1. What produces the barking cough?

2. Should the responding EMTs examine inside Adam's mouth? Why or why not?

Critical Thinking 3: Read the following scenario and then answer the questions.

Mr. Williamson called for EMS fairly often. He had a history of COPD and often found that he couldn't breathe well, even when taking his medication as prescribed. This time was far worse, however. By the time the EMTs had arrived, Mr. Williamson could hardly breathe at all!

While Jason began an initial assessment, Beth attempted to obtain a history. Mr. Williamson found it difficult to answer questions. Beth did discover that he had been exposed to some irritating vapors from a construction site nearby. Although it was quite cold out that day, the previous evening had been rather warm, and Mr. Williamson had kept his window open.

1. Should the EMTs administer oxygen to Mr. Williamson? Why or why not?

2. How should the EMTs prepare Mr. Williamson for transport?

CHAPTER 28
Chest Pain

EMT-Bs are frequently called to the scene of a patient experiencing chest pain. The accurate assessment and quick management of a patient with chest pain is the key to patient survival.

Definitions: Read each definition. Write the correct word or phrase on the line.

1. Pain produced by injured or dying heart muscle ____________________
2. Deposits of fat on the walls of arteries ____________________
3. Bulging veins of the neck (abbreviation) ____________________
4. Elevated BP ____________________
5. A blood clot ____________________
6. Arteries that provide blood to the heart muscle ____________________
7. Shock produced when the heart fails as a pump ____________________
8. The heart muscle ____________________
9. Blockage ____________________
10. Abnormally fast heart rate ____________________
11. Excessive perspiration due to stress or pain ____________________
12. Abdominal area just below the sternum ____________________
13. Abnormally slow heart rate ____________________
14. Circulation of oxygen and nutrients to cells ____________________

Identification: List 11 risk factors for cardiovascular disease. Place the risk factors in the correct column as modifiable or nonmodifiable.

Modifiable risk factors	**Nonmodifiable risk factors**
____________________	____________________
____________________	____________________
____________________	____________________
____________________	____________________
____________________	____________________
____________________	____________________
____________________	____________________

Labeling: Label the systemic and pulmonary circulations on the diagram.

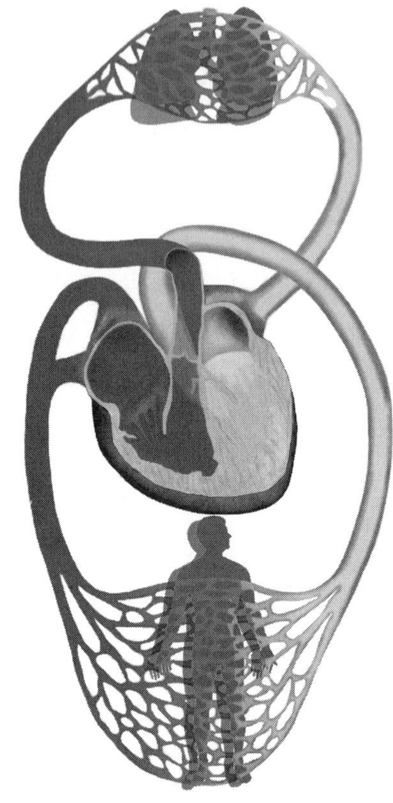

Identification: Read the common description given and write on the line the sign or symptom described.

1. Viselike ____________________
2. Toothache ____________________
3. Heartburn ____________________
4. Not enough oxygen ____________________
5. No energy ____________________
6. Cannot catch breath ____________________
7. Dizzy ____________________
8. Pressure ____________________
9. Numbness/heaviness ____________________
10. Indigestion ____________________

True or False: Read each statement and decide if it is true or false. Place T or F on the line before each statement.

1. _____ In assessing a patient with chest pain, it is not important to know what the patient was doing.
2. _____ Loss of consciousness is associated with cardiac problems.
3. _____ Neck and jaw pain are associated with cardiac chest pain.
4. _____ An older patient without a cardiac history is not likely having an MI.
5. _____ Cardiac pain always radiates to the left shoulder.
6. _____ Positional chest pain is highly indicative of a cardiac event.

7. ______ The therapeutic goal for a patient with chest pain is to reduce the pain by 50%.
8. ______ The EMT-B must ask about over-the-counter medications taken for pain.
9. ______ It is relatively uncommon for a young person to have a heart attack.
10. ______ Illicit drugs may lead to heart attacks in young adults.

Ordering: Place the following actions in the order in which they should be performed for a physical assessment of a patient complaining of chest pain. Put a numeral 1 before the first action, a 2 before the next, and so on.

______ Complete a focused physical exam

______ Assess the airway

______ Obtain baseline vital signs

______ Get a SAMPLE history

______ Survey the scene for safety

______ Check circulation

______ Note general impression

______ Assess breathing adequacy

Short Answer: Read each question. Think about the information presented in your text, and then answer each question with one or two sentences.

1. Why is it important for the EMT to provide early cardiac care?

2. Where does the heart muscle obtain its oxygen and nutrients?

3. Is it important for the EMT to be able to distinguish the diagnosis of angina from acute myocardial infarction?

Critical Thinking: Read the following scenario and then answer the questions.

Ambulance One responded to a call for a man with chest pressure. Mr. Stevens, 62 years old, had his wife call 9-1-1 after experiencing 2 hours of discomfort.

1. What are the components of the focused history and physical exam that should be performed on Mr. Stevens?

Mr. Stevens had a prescription for nitroglycerine. The EMTs assisted him in taking the medication.

2. What assessments must be made after Mr. Stevens takes the medication?

Five minutes after taking his nitroglycerine, Mr. Stevens complained of feeling dizzy. His blood pressure was 80/40.

3. How should the EMTs manage Mr. Stevens now?

CHAPTER 29
Cardiac Arrest

In the not too distant past, cardiac arrest was a death sentence. However, advances in medicine and technology have made out-of-hospital arrest reversal more likely. EMTs, carrying special devices called automatic external defibrillators, are able to provide definitive care to the cardiac arrest victim.

Definitions: Write the definitions of the following terms.

1. defibrillation
2. dysrhythmia
3. electrocardiogram
4. automaticity
5. rhythm
6. sudden cardiac death
7. chain of survival
8. public access defibrillation
9. artificial pacemaker
10. all clear command

Labeling: Label the sinoatrial node, the atrioventricular node, the bundle of His, the right and left bundle branches, the AV bundle, and the Purkinje fibers in the figure below.

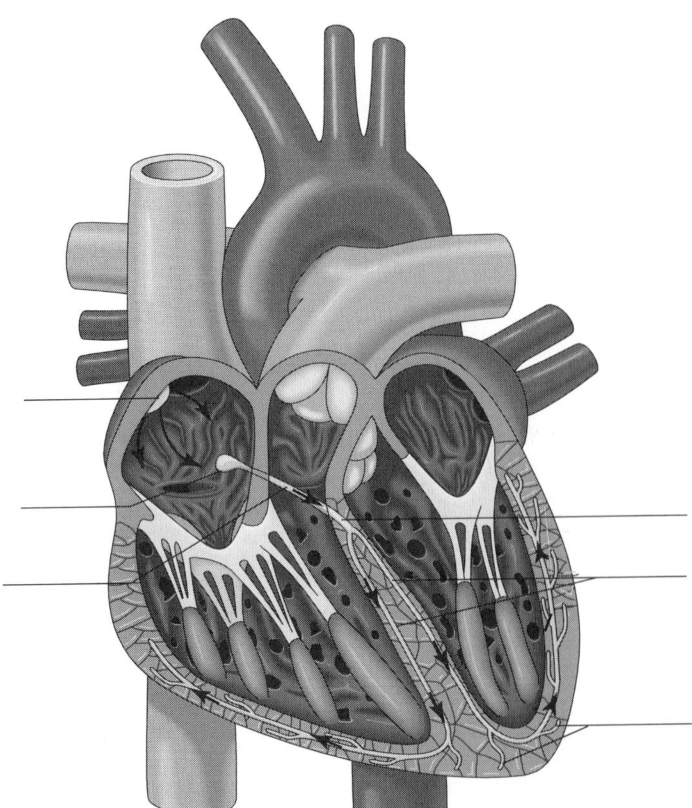

Identification: Identify each of the cardiac rhythms in Figures A, B, C, and D. Write the correct interpretation in the space provided.

A.

B.

C.

D.

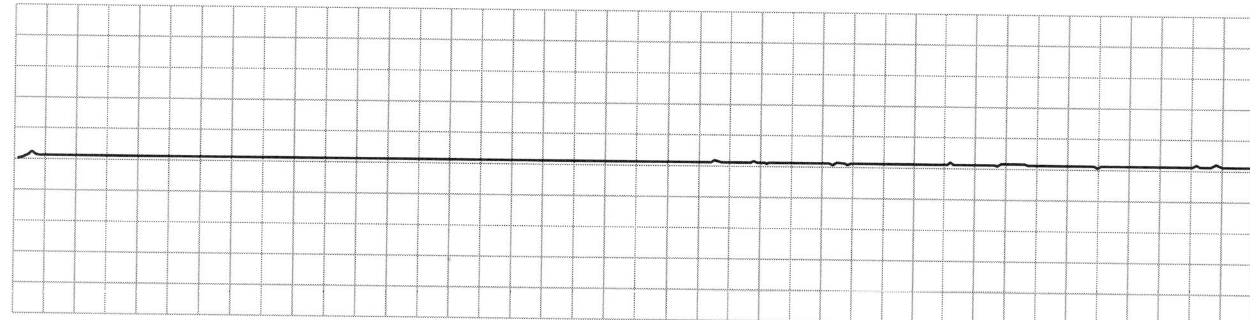

A.

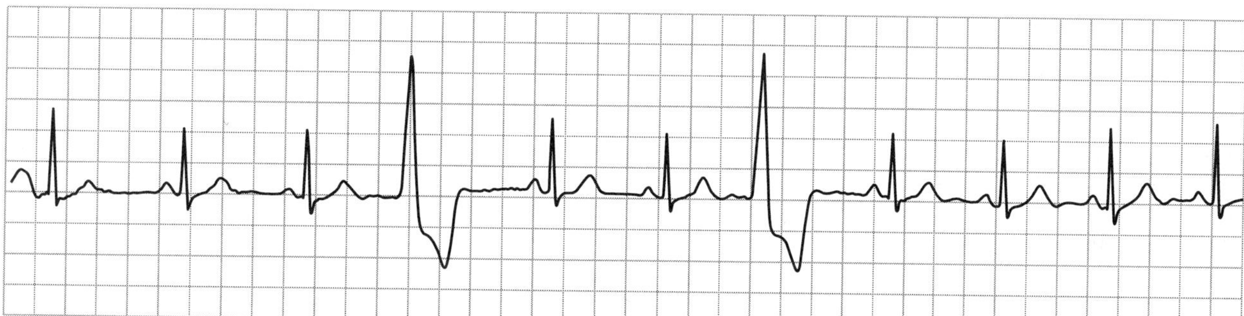

B.

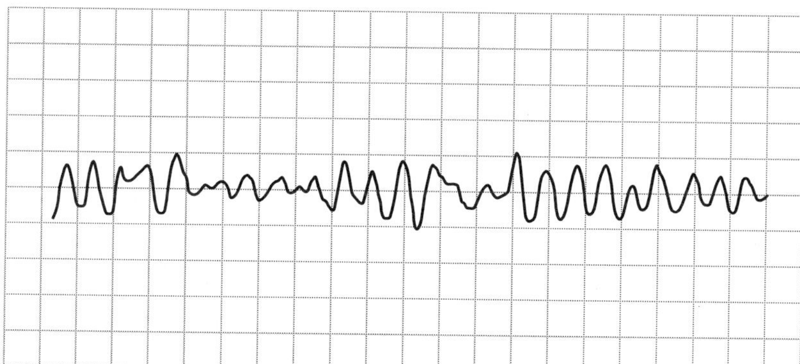

C.

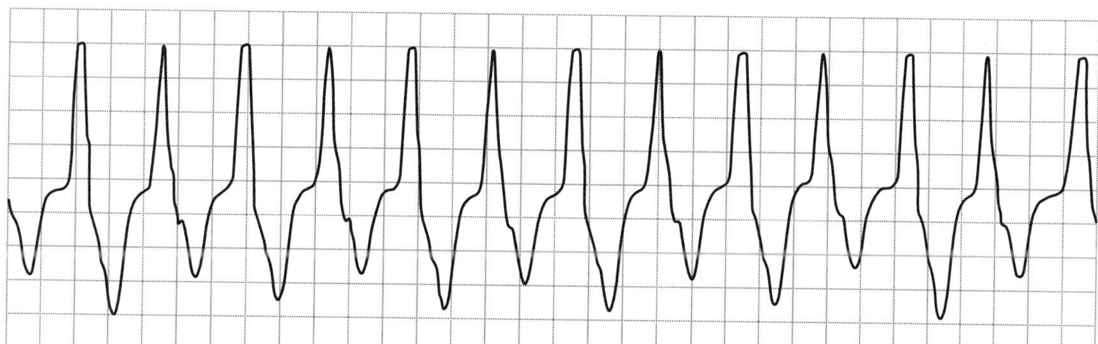

D.

Ordering: Place the following assessment in order by placing a numeral 1 before the first thing to be done, 2 before the next, and so on.

_____ Open airway

_____ BSI/scene safety

_____ Check for carotid pulse

_____ Observe for chest rise

_____ Check responsiveness

Ordering: Place the following management techniques in order by placing a numeral a numeral 1 before the first thing to be done, 2 before the next, and so on.

_____ Turn on AED and stop touching the patient

_____ Reanalyze/reassess

_____ Analyze rhythm

_____ Assess patient

_____ Apply patches/cable

_____ Clear patient for shock

_____ Press "shock" button

Identification: Read each of the following phrases. Decide if it is an indication for use of an AED or a contraindication. Write "indication" or "contraindication" on the line in front of each phrase.

1. ____________________ Complaining of chest pain
2. ____________________ Thrashing
3. ____________________ Pulseless
4. ____________________ Airway blocked
5. ____________________ No carotid pulse
6. ____________________ No radial pulse while crying
7. ____________________ P on AVPU
8. ____________________ 5 years old
9. ____________________ mortal injuries
10. ____________________ pulseless, apneic, weighing 75 lb

True or False: Read each sentence regarding safety and determine if it is true or false. Write T or F on the line before each statement.

1. _____ Using paddles for defibrillation gives the EMT better control of the procedure.
2. _____ Chest compressions can mimic ventricular fibrillation.
3. _____ Defibrillation should take place in a moving ambulance.
4. _____ "All clear" means that persons may touch the patient again.
5. _____ Do not defibrillate a patient who is in a puddle of water.
6. _____ It is acceptable for an EMT to override the suggestions of the AED.
7. _____ Be sure no one is touching the stretcher carriage during defibrillation.

8. ______ The operator of the AED is responsible for crew, bystander, and patient safety.
9. ______ Perform a head-to-toe sweep before discharging the AED.
10. ______ Move the AED pads away from an implanted pacemaker.
11. ______ Move a patient off a metal fire escape before defibrillating.
12. ______ Defib pads are effective when partially in contact with skin.

Short Answer: Read each question. Think about the information presented in your text, and then answer each question with one or two sentences.

1. List two reasons that EMTs should use an AED specifically designed for children on those patients younger than nine years old or weighing less than 25 kg (55 pounds).

2. Why would the EMT still have patients to care for after someone is declared dead?

Critical Thinking 1: Read the following scenario and then answer the questions.

MaryLou and Chris arrived at the home of Mr. Roberts, a 50-year-old man who had collapsed in his front yard. His wife and daughter were performing CPR.

1. What should MaryLou and Chris do first?

2. Describe the necessary care for Mr. Roberts.

After the fourth shock, the AED read NO SHOCK ADVISED.

3. What should the EMTs do now?

Following ALS interventions by paramedics, Mr. Roberts is declared dead.

4. What care is necessary now?

Critical Thinking 2: Read the following scenario and then answer the questions.

The EMT supervisor arrived at the scene of a "cardiac problem." Bev and Joe were caring for a 62-year-old female who was complaining of severe chest pain. They had placed her in a comfortable position, applied oxygen, and were in the process of applying the AED patches.

1. Do you agree with the care that was being provided?

2. If you were the EMT supervisor, how would you have handled this situation?

Chapter 29 Skill Sheet

Student Name ______________________ Date ____________

Skill 29-1: Operation of an Automated External Defibrillator

Equipment Needed:

1. Automated external defibrillator
2. Personal protective clothing

Yes: ❑ Reteach: ❑ Return: ❑ Instructor initials: ________

Step 1: Confirm that the patient is in cardiac arrest.

Yes: ❑ Reteach: ❑ Return: ❑ Instructor initials: ________

Step 2: Apply the electrode pads to the anterior chest wall, one to the apex of the heart at the lower left rib cage, and the other to the right sternal border below the clavicle.

Yes: ❑ Reteach: ❑ Return: ❑ Instructor initials: ________

Step 3: Turn the power on the AED while calling *all clear*. Ensure that no one is touching the patient.

Yes: ❑ Reteach: ❑ Return: ❑ Instructor initials: ________

Step 4: Press the *analyze* button and press the *shock* button, as advised. Again, ensure that no one is touching the patient.

Yes: ❑ Reteach: ❑ Return: ❑ Instructor initials: ________

Step 5: After the series of shocks have been performed, check for the presence or absence of a pulse. If the pulse is absent, CPR must be continued for another minute. If the patient's pulse returns, check for breathing. If the patient's pulse does not return, then another round of shocks may be indicated.

Yes: ❑ Reteach: ❑ Return: ❑ Instructor initials: ________

NREMT Skill Sheet

Cardiac Arrest Management/AED

Start Time: ______________________

Stop Time: ______________________ **Date:** ______________

Candidate's Name: ______________________________________

Evaluator's Name: ______________________________________

	Points Possible	Points Awarded
ASSESSMENT		
Takes, or verbalizes, body substance isolation precautions	1	
Briefly questions the rescuer about arrest events	1	
Directs rescuer to stop CPR	1	
Verifies absence of spontaneous pulse (skill station examiner states "no pulse")	1	
Directs resumption of CPR	1	
Turns on defibrillator power	1	
Attaches automated defibrillator to the patient	1	
Directs rescuer to stop CPR and ensures all individuals are clear of the patient	1	
Initiates analysis of the rhythm	1	
Delivers shock (up to three successive shocks)	1	
Verifies absence of spontaneous pulse (skill station examiner states "no pulse")	1	
TRANSITION		
Directs resumption of CPR	1	
Gathers additional information about arrest event	1	
Confirms effectiveness of CPR (ventilation and compressions)	1	
INTEGRATION		
Verbalizes or directs insertion of a simple airway adjunct (oral/nasal airway)	1	
Ventilates, or directs ventilation of, the patient	1	
Assures high concentration of oxygen is delivered to the patient	1	
Assures CPR continues without unnecessary/prolonged interruption	1	
Re-evaluates patient/CPR in approximately one minute	1	
Repeats defibrillator sequence	1	
TRANSPORTATION		
Verbalizes transportation of patient	1	
Total:	21	

Critical Criteria

_______ Did not take, or verbalize, body substance isolation precautions

_______ Did not evaluate the need for immediate use of the AED

_______ Did not direct initiation/resumption of ventilation/compressions at appropriate times

_______ Did not assure all individuals were clear of patient before delivering each shock

_______ Did not operate the AED properly (inability to deliver shock)

_______ Prevented the defibrillator from delivering indicated stacked shocks

CHAPTER 30
Altered Mental Status

A patient may act confused, disoriented, or may "just not be acting right." The behavior may be due to illness, injury, or disease and is called altered mental status. Several potentially dangerous medical conditions can create this, and the EMT must understand them and their management.

Matching: Match each word or term with its definition

1. _____ aura
2. _____ AEIOU TIPS
3. _____ altered mental state
4. _____ Alzheimer's disease
5. _____ anticonvulsant
6. _____ diabetes mellitus
7. _____ diabetic coma
8. _____ diet-controlled diabetes
9. _____ gestational diabetes
10. _____ grand mal seizure
11. _____ insulin shock
12. _____ amnesia
13. _____ status epilepticus
14. _____ petit mal seizure
15. _____ oral hypoglycemic

a. one continuous seizure
b. old term for generalized seizure
c. diabetes occurring in pregnancy
d. old term for partial seizure
e. disease in which the pancreas fails
f. blood sugar control through eating habits
g. drug to control seizures
h. a progressive deterioration of brain function
i. drug that stimulates insulin production
j. unconscious patient with high blood sugar
k. a change in behavior
l. a way to remember the causes of AMS
m. failure to remember what happened
n. warning sign at the onset of a seizure
o. a low blood sugar

Correcting: Each of the following statements is false. Rewrite it as a correct statement.

1. A person experiencing a change in behavior that may be due to illness or injury is having a psychiatric crisis.
2. A person who fails to remember what just happened is anaerobic.
3. Hypoglycemia is a lack of oxygen in the blood.
4. Diabetes mellitus occurs when the liver fails to produce sufficient insulin.
5. Excessive thirst is called polyuria.
6. The development of hyperglycemia is a sudden event, often occurring over minutes to an hour.
7. When the body cannot use sugar for energy, it uses ketoacids instead.
8. Kussmaul's respirations are slow and shallow.
9. Insulin shock results from excessive sugar in the blood.
10. A patient experiencing a low blood sugar will have warm, dry, flushed skin.
11. The cause of epilepsy is well-defined.
12. In a seizure affecting the whole brain, just a portion of the body is affected.

13. An origin is an odor or flash of light or sound that precedes certain seizures.
14. The postictal phase of a seizure occurs when the body stiffens.
15. Managing a seizing patient includes restraining the body.

Short Answer: Read each question. Think about the information presented in your text, and then answer each question with one or two sentences.

1. Why will the brain "malfunction" when glucose is not available?

2. How can a person have diabetes mellitus and still produce insulin?

3. What is epilepsy? Name causes of seizures besides epilepsy.

4. Can someone have a seizure and still remain standing?

Listing: List the necessary steps for a fingerstick glucose test. (You may or may not need all 16 lines.)

1. __________
2. __________
3. __________
4. __________
5. __________
6. __________
7. __________
8. __________
9. __________
10. __________
11. __________
12. __________
13. __________
14. __________
15. __________
16. __________

Critical Thinking 1: Read the following scenario and then answer the questions.

Bethany and Dean arrived on the scene of a bicycle accident to find a middle-aged man lying on the sidewalk next to his bike. Witnesses state that the man was "all over the place" just prior to taking a tumble. The witnesses could not figure out why the guy fell over; he didn't hit anything, and nothing was close to hit him.

Dean checked for responsiveness and took C-spine precautions to ensure that the neck and back stayed still. The man did not respond to Dean when he called to him. Bethany removed the bike helmet and completed an initial assessment. While looking for any signs of bleeding, she found a medic alert tag reading diabetes mellitus. No injuries were found during Bethany's exam. The man never responded to the touch or movements during the exam.

1. What do you think may have caused this incident?

2. How should the EMTs manage it?

3. Is the use of oral glucose indicated here? Why or why not?

Critical Thinking 2: Read the following scenario and then answer the questions.

The school nurse called EMS for a child actively seizing in the gymnasium. Upon arrival, Nora and Rich found a 10-year-old child lying on the mat beneath a climbing wall. The child was very still and snoring. The nurse related that the child had no significant medical history and was on no medications.

1. Name some likely causes of the child's current condition.

2. What safety precautions should the EMTs take to protect themselves and the child?

3. What measures must the EMTs take immediately during the initial assessment?

4. Is the use of oral glucose indicated here? Why or why not?

5. Is the use of oxygen indicated here? Why or why not?

Review glucose administration in Chapter 26.

CHAPTER 31
Stroke

Early identification of the possibility of stroke and appropriate decision making on the part of the EMT can have a significant impact on the morbidity and mortality associated with this condition.

Matching: Match each word or term with its definition.

1. _____ receptive aphasia
2. _____ dysarthria
3. _____ expressive aphasia
4. _____ facial droop
5. _____ pronator drift

a. clear speech but use of incorrect words
b. inability to hold arms out and keep them up
c. the face doesn't move symmetrically
d. inability to understand what is spoken
e. difficulty in producing clear speech

Definitions: Write the definitions of the following terms.

1. stroke ______________________________
2. hemorrhagic stroke ______________________________
3. ischemic stroke ______________________________
4. cerebrovascular accident (CVA) ______________________________
5. transient ischemic attack (TIA) ______________________________
6. embolus ______________________________
7. thrombus ______________________________

Labeling: Label the infarct region and the penumbra. Underneath each label, state whether the region can be saved or not.

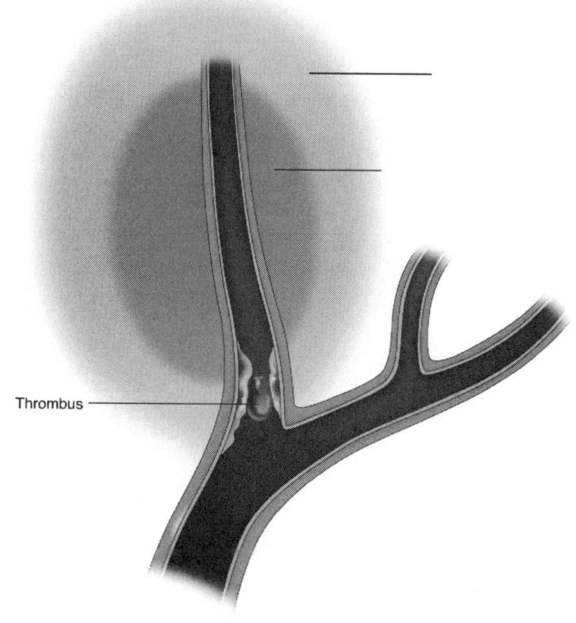

Listing: List the three components of the Cincinnati Prehospital Stroke Scale in the first column. Then list the normal response for each component in the second column. In the third column, list the abnormal response, and in the fourth column, describe a method that the EMT can use to assess the component.

Component	Normal	Abnormal	Way to assess

Identification: Name six other conditions that may present strokelike symptoms.

1. ______________________________
2. ______________________________
3. ______________________________
4. ______________________________
5. ______________________________
6. ______________________________

Short Answer: Read the question. Think about the information presented in your text, and then answer the question with one or two sentences.

1. What treatments can the EMT offer to a patient with strokelike symptoms?

Critical Thinking 1: Read the following scenario and then answer the questions.

Debra and Brian were called to the home of Mr. Mantelli. His wife was frantic! She states that he was watching TV and suddenly dropped his glass and began mumbling unintelligible words. She called 9-1-1 right away because she thought he was having a heart attack!

1. What are some likely explanations for Mr. Mantelli's symptoms?

Exam shows that Mr. Mantelli has an open airway, is breathing well and without difficulty, and has strong distal pulses. His blood pressure is 136/86; pulse is 72 and regular; respirations are 18 and nonlabored; skin is warm and dry. When asked to smile, Mr. Mantelli looks as if one side of his face is smiling and the other side is scowling. He cannot hold his arms out in front of him, and he cannot speak clearly.

2. What treatments should Debra and Brian provide for Mr. Mantelli?

3. What should they tell Mrs. Mantelli?

Critical Thinking 2: Read the following scenario and then answer the questions.

Cindy was saying hello to her new partner, Kim, when the tones sounded. They were sent to the local fitness center for a middle-aged man who was slurring his speech. His friend states that he took his Imitrex today and then came to the fitness center at his friend's insistence.

1. Name some likely causes of the man's current condition.

2. What assessments should Kim and Cindy make during their physical exam?

The man stated that he smelled coffee, didn't feel well, and sat down. His speech was so unclear that Kim had difficulty figuring out what was said. He also had pronator (arm) drift.

3. How should the EMTs treat this man?

After the EMTs had brought him to a hospital, the doctor told them that this man had a complicated migraine headache and that they had done a good job.

4. Explain to Kim and Cindy how they could be wrong on their diagnosis and still had done a good job.

CHAPTER 32
Abnormal Behavior

Mental illness is any disorder that affects the mind and is exhibited in a person's behavior. EMTs are less interested in the specific diagnoses of mental illness than in the behaviors that would generate an EMS call.

Matching: Match each word or term with its definition.

1. _____ anxiety disorder	a.	sudden, erratic behavioral change
2. _____ dementia	b.	hyperactive irrational behavior
3. _____ hallucination	c.	psychological need for a drug
4. _____ addiction	d.	unreal sensations or perceptions
5. _____ withdrawal symptoms	e.	nonphysical disorder that impairs brain function
6. _____ suicide	f.	voluntary taking of own life
7. _____ mental illness	g.	gradual loss of ability to think
8. _____ dependency	h.	side effects of stopping some drugs
9. _____ excited delirium	i.	abnormal response to stress
10. _____ delirium	j.	physical need for a drug

Identification: Read each description and write the type of hallucination on the line.

1. ______________________ Sense of spiders walking on the skin
2. ______________________ God said to steal an item
3. ______________________ A mirage
4. ______________________ Sense of people talking about your clothes
5. ______________________ Perception that a clock is chiming
6. ______________________ Sense that Mom said to damage the car
7. ______________________ Sense that someone is touching your arm
8. ______________________ Sense that a dog is sitting there

Identification: Read each definition and write the correct name of the restraint device or action on the line.

1. ______________________ Holding or tying the arms and legs
2. ______________________ Heavy-duty, commercial wrist and ankle devices
3. ______________________ Totally encapsulating a patient
4. ______________________ Layering linens around a patient
5. ______________________ Planned, orderly method of subduing someone
6. ______________________ Suffocation resulting from an inability to breathe
7. ______________________ Minimum effort needed to confine a person
8. ______________________ Demonstration of determination
9. ______________________ Confined in order to protect the patient from harming himself

Sorting: Read each behavior listed and decide if the behavior is a behavioral emergency. Place a checkmark in front of each instance that is a behavioral emergency. For each that is a behavioral emergency, describe how the EMT should handle the situation.

1. _____ A young mother is crying after the death of her infant.

2. _____ A teenager is threatening to shoot himself after getting a bad grade.

3. _____ A young man is crying loudly after he dropped his soda.

4. _____ A middle-aged woman is upset that she is having breathing difficulties.

5. _____ An elderly man is afraid that he will die if he enters a hospital.

6. _____ A young man threatens to kill all people who wear uniforms.

7. _____ A middle-aged man expresses anger that his wife just died.

8. _____ A newly arrived immigrant cannot follow a person's directions.

9. _____ A young man is upset after the saw he was using sliced his hand.

10. _____ A teenaged girl states she is going to stab all the snakes in the room.

True or False: Read each statement and decide if it is true or false. Place T or F on the line before each statement.

1. ______ You should only enter an unsafe scene during daylight hours.
2. ______ Always wear gloves when touching an object on a crime scene.
3. ______ Continually alert the dispatcher to what you are doing when approaching a potentially violent person.
4. ______ When walking with other EMTs, proceed side by side.
5. ______ An EMT can detect anger by the patient's posture.
6. ______ Rapid eye movements may indicate panic.
7. ______ The EMT should have an escape plan ready at all times.
8. ______ When gathering a history, the EMT should stand very close to the patient.
9. ______ Only one EMT should question the patient.
10. ______ The EMT should always speak louder than the patient.

Short Answer: Read each question. Think about the information presented in your text, and then answer each question with one or two sentences.

1. Why is an adult patient experiencing a behavioral crisis not permitted to refuse restraints?

2. What is the minimum number of people required for a takedown? Why?

3. Once the patient is placed in the ambulance, where should the EMT sit to provide care? What tasks can be completed from this vantage point?

4. How often should pulses, movement, and sensation be checked in a restrained patient?

Critical Thinking 1: Read the scenario and then answer the questions.

Geoff and Sandy responded to a call at Corner Ice Cream for a man acting strangely. It was not difficult to locate the man, as a large crowd of people had gathered in the parking lot. When they arrived, the man seemed to be mumbling words and striking out at thin air. Several of the onlookers were laughing and jeering at him, calling him an old drunk. Sandy requested a police unit to the scene and when it arrived, Sandy and the officer carefully approached the patient. Geoff and the second officer watched the group of onlookers. The man was unable to answer questions; he just kept mumbling words. Neither Sandy nor the officer was able to detect any odor of an alcoholic beverage on him. Just when the man struck out at thin air, Sandy spied a medic alert tag detailing a history of diabetes.

1. Is this a behavioral emergency?

2. Is it likely that the cause of this situation is organic?

3. How should Geoff and Sandy proceed in the care of this man?

Critical Thinking 2: Read the scenario and then answer the questions.

Security at the arena called for EMS to evaluate a man whose behavior seemed bizarre. Janie and Ralph responded, taking care to evaluate scene safety. The man was seated on the floor outside the men's lavatory. Every few minutes he would scream out that he "hated them and would jump and take them all with him."

1. Is there a behavioral emergency here?
2. How should Janie and Ralph approach this patient?

Janie spoke first to the patient. He told her that the voices kept telling him to do things, and he hated them. The voices, he said, told him that Janie was there to hurt him.

3. How should Janie react to the idea that she was trying to hurt the patient?
4. What should she say next?
5. Should Ralph speak with the patient? Why or why not?

The man agreed to go to the hospital. The security guard accompanied Janie in the back of the ambulance.

CHAPTER 33
Abdominal Pain

Abdominal pain is the most common complaint of patients arriving at the emergency department. It is important for prehospital providers to understand the potential for serious illness when a patient complains of abdominal pain.

Matching: Match each word or term with its definition.

1. _____ abdominal aortic aneurysm
2. _____ appendicitis
3. _____ bowel obstruction
4. _____ cholecystitis
5. _____ diverticulitis
6. _____ ectopic pregnancy
7. _____ esophageal varices
8. _____ gastroenteritis
9. _____ pancreatitis
10. _____ pyelonephritis
11. _____ renal stone
12. _____ ulcer

a. infection in the large bowel causing left quadrant pain
b. inflammation of the organ which secretes digestive enzymes into the duodenum
c. a weakened area in the vessel wall that balloons into the abdomen
d. kidney infection
e. a viral illness causing vomiting and diarrhea
f. often characterized by right lower quadrant pain
g. solid material that may block a ureter
h. block in the intestines which leads to bloating
i. infection of the gallbladder
j. erosion of the stomach lining
k. implantation outside of the uterus
l. dilated veins in the tube between the mouth and stomach

Definitions: Write the definitions of the following terms.

1. hematochezia ______________________________
2. hemetemesis ______________________________
3. jaundice ______________________________
4. melena ______________________________

Listing: List the organs found in each region or system.

1. Abdominal region

2. Genitourinary

3. Hematologic system

Short Answer: From your textbook, give three ways in which abdominal problems can lead to shock.

Critical Thinking: Read the following scenario and then answer the questions.

Donte and Genna answered a call to Schermerhorn Road. Their patient, Kevin Smythe, was a 37-year-old man who was complaining of left-sided flank pain that seemed to circle around to his stomach and groin. Donte gathered a history while Genna applied oxygen. Mr. Smythe said that his pain had begun about two hours earlier but now he was vomiting and "just couldn't take it any longer." He also reported that the oxygen had not helped at all.

1. What is the likely cause of Mr. Smythe's pain?

2. What should Genna and Donte do next?

3. What care do you anticipate for Mr. Smythe during his transport to the hospital?

CHAPTER 34
Environmental Emergencies

In addition to exposure to the elements, water, and altitude, the EMT must be familiar with other emergencies created by outdoor activities, such as lightning strikes and bites.

Matching: Match each word or term with its definition.

1. _____ chilblains	a.	skin freezing
2. _____ trench foot	b.	life-threatening heat illness
3. _____ frostnip	c.	joint pain occurring after a rapid ascent
4. _____ frostbite	d.	swelling of the brain from hypoxia at high altitudes
5. _____ hypothermia	e.	a reversible effect of breathing nitrogen
6. _____ heat cramps	f.	causes rupture of the alveoli
7. _____ heat exhaustion	g.	submersion not resulting in death within 24 hours
8. _____ heat stroke	h.	core body temperature below 95°F
9. _____ bends	i.	inflammed area due to chronic cool and dampness
10. _____ air embolism	j.	cough and dyspnea associated with high altitudes
11. _____ HACE	k.	painful muscle spasms from loss of fluids
12. _____ HAPE	l.	tissue injury from chronic wet conditions
13. _____ nitrogen narcosis	m.	mild, generalized heat sickness with dehydration
14. _____ near-drowning	n.	air in a vessel resulting in a blockage of blood flow
15. _____ pulmonary over-pressurization syndrome	o.	local skin injury from freezing weather

Sorting: Read each action and then place each in the category describing the specific type of heat loss.

Removing your sweater in a cool room	Entering a meat cooler
Sitting on cold rocks	Sweating
Breathing	Swimming in a cold lake
Sitting in front of a fan	Standing in the wind
Turning on the air conditioner in the house	Lying on a waterbed heated to 70°F

Radiation	**Convection**	**Conduction**	**Evaporation**

Identification: Place an X in front of those conditions that place persons at greater risk for hypothermia.

1. _____ diabetes mellitus
2. _____ adolescence
3. _____ heart disease
4. _____ multiple medications
5. _____ isolated broken wrist
6. _____ generalized infection
7. _____ burns
8. _____ sprained ankle
9. _____ thyroid condition
10. _____ head injury
11. _____ shock
12. _____ infected tooth
13. _____ spinal cord injury

Treatments: For each of the following conditions, list the management.

Local cold injuries

Hypothermia

Heat cramps

Heat exhaustion

Heat stroke

Snake bites

Sorting: Place an X in front of those signs or symptoms seen in hypothermia.

1. _____ poor coordination
2. _____ flushing
3. _____ nausea
4. _____ slurred speech
5. _____ poor judgment
6. _____ slow pulse
7. _____ pale skin
8. _____ stomach cramps
9. _____ mood changes
10. _____ decreased sensation
11. _____ muscle cramps
12. _____ itching

Identification: Which of these are active measures of rewarming, and which are passive? Place the answer on the line in front of each.

1. ____________________ heat packs to groin
2. ____________________ blankets
3. ____________________ hot water bottles to arms
4. ____________________ shelter from wind
5. ____________________ removing wet clothing
6. ____________________ hot drinks
7. ____________________ heating pads
8. ____________________ hat on head

Ordering: Place the following methods for water rescue in order of priority, putting a numeral 1 before the first step, 2 before the next, and so on.

_____	row	_____	go
_____	reach	_____	throw

Listing: List the types of incidents (injuries) that occur at each phase of diving.

Descent

Ascent

Fill in the Blank: Complete the following paragraph regarding lightning strikes.

Lightning strikes are divided into ____________________ and ____________________ injuries. With lesser injuries, the common symptoms include ____________________, ____________________, and short-term memory difficulties. A large percentage of people suffer ruptured ____________________. They may also suffer ____________________ trauma. The EMT should ____________________ the patient to prevent any further injuries.

In other people, the electricity produces a shock that stops ____________________ electrical activity and a full arrest occurs. Even if the heart resumes function, the ____________________ may continue to malfunction, preventing ____________________ effort and resulting in hypoxia.

The first priority in the management of a victim of a lightning strike is ____________________ ____________________.

Short Answer: Read each question. Think about the information presented in your text, and then answer each question with one or two sentences.

1. Name two major ways in which the body loses heat.

2. Describe how the body generates heat.

3. Describe two ways in which the body conserves heat.

4. Give two reasons why the elderly and very young cannot protect themselves against the extremes of heat and cold.

5. Explain how afterdrop occurs.

6. Name the complications of near-drowning.

7. How are diving emergencies related to drowning emergencies?

8. Why is oxygen indicated for managing mountain sickness?

Critical Thinking 1: Read the following scenario and then answer the questions.

Jessie and Anne responded to a call at a construction site for a man who had fallen off a scaffold. Upon their arrival, they found one man lying on wet ground and not moving and three more confused and dazed. The foreman told them it was the most incredible scene he had ever witnessed. The four men were about 8 feet up when a freak storm hit. The rain was blinding, and the thunder resonated through the site. When it was over, Jay, his best employee, lay on the ground, and Jimmy, Ron, and Eric were acting strangely.

1. What is the likely cause of this situation?

2. What is their first priority with this call?

3. Who should the EMTs care for first?

4. What other injuries must the EMTs be concerned with?

Critical Thinking 2: Read the following scenario and then answer the questions.

Debra and Brandon were sent to the home of Mrs. Miller, an 80-year-old woman living alone. The mailman had reported that Mrs. Miller was "not herself" today.

As they approached the home, a single-family bungalow in a quiet section of town, they remarked on the sudden cold snap. It was only September, but it seemed more like December in the Northeast. The mailman was waiting outside the home for the EMTs, and he commented on how well Mrs. Miller had seemed yesterday. Brandon noticed that all first-floor windows in the house were open.

Mrs. Miller was sitting on her couch. Her speech was slurred and she seemed unable to move easily. Her arms and torso were cold to the touch.

1. What do the EMTs know about this event?

2. How should they proceed?

Critical Thinking 3: Read the following scenario and then answer the questions.

It was late October, and George realized he was late in bringing wood in for the stove. While stacking wood next to the woodpile, he felt a pinch on his leg. Not being a man to complain, he continued working until the swelling became too bad. Now, he had severe stomach pain and a very weak feeling.

1. What likely happened to George?

2. How should the EMTs manage care for him?

3. Should George be seen at a hospital?

CHAPTER 35
Poisoning and Allergic Reactions

Exposure to substances with deadly ingredients can cause predictable or unpredictable reactions. It is important for the EMT to be familiar with the concepts of poisonings and allergic reactions, and understand their priorities and management.

Matching: Match each word or term with its definition.

1.	_____	allergen	a.	hives
2.	_____	anaphylaxis	b.	prevents the absorption of some substances
3.	_____	overdose	c.	amount of time that eyes should be flushed
4.	_____	stridor	d.	causes activation of immune system
5.	_____	urticaria	e.	time when an allergic reaction normally starts
6.	_____	reaction	f.	serious allergic reaction that leads to shock
7.	_____	poison control	g.	often indicative of vocal chord swelling
8.	_____	charcoal	h.	response to allergen
9.	_____	20 minutes	i.	resource regarding various substances
10.	_____	30 minutes	j.	often deliberate overexposure to drug

Definitions: Write the definitions of the following terms.

1. allergic reaction

2. epinephrine

3. ingestion

4. inhalation

5. injected

6. absorbed

7. poisoning

Identification: Identify each of the following as caused by injected, inhaled, absorbed, or ingested poisons.

1. Spider bite ______________________________
2. Bee sting ______________________________
3. Drain cleaner ______________________________
4. Car exhaust ______________________________
5. Chlorine gas ______________________________
6. Poison ivy ______________________________
7. Chemical fire extinguisher ______________________________
8. Mace/pepper spray ______________________________
9. Alcohol ______________________________
10. Marijuana ______________________________

True or False: Read each statement and decide if it is true or false. Place T or F on the line before each statement.

1. _____ Activated charcoal should be given only within one to two hours of ingesting a substance.
2. _____ Activated charcoal should be used only with patients who have ingested caustic substances.
3. _____ Patients who are unconscious should be given activated charcoal.
4. _____ Activated charcoal is given in doses of 10 to 20 g for an adult.
5. _____ Adrenalin is another term for epinephrine.
6. _____ An EpiPen gives a dose of 0.3 to 0.5 mg.
7. _____ Stridor is an indication for use of activated charcoal.

Completion: Complete the following drug card for activated charcoal.

Generic name activated charcoal

Trade name

Indication

Contraindication

Dose

Route

Completion: Complete the following drug card for an epinephrine auto-injector.

Generic name Epinephrine

Trade name

Indication

Contraindication

Dose

Route

Short Answer: Read each question. Think about the information presented in your text, and then answer each question with one or two sentences.

1. How do the assessment findings differ between a mild and a severe allergic reaction?

2. What are the signs that a patient with an allergic reaction is worsening?

Critical Thinking 1: Read the following scenario and then answer the questions.

An EMT performed CPR on a man's bare chest without using gloves. He later found that he had a pasty substance on his hands. The patient's wife stated that the patient uses nitroglycerin paste. The EMT is now feeling dizzy and lightheaded.

1. What is the route of exposure?

2. How should the EMTs manage it?

Critical Thinking 2: Read the following scenario and then answer the questions.

Meredith was mowing her lawn and disturbed a wasp's nest. She was stung repeatedly and stated, "I can't breathe." She had a high-pitched sound coming from her breathing.

1. What is the route of exposure?

2. How should the EMTs manage it?

Critical Thinking 3: Read the following scenario and then answer the questions.

Aimee was expecting company this evening and decided to give her apartment a good cleaning. To ensure it was clean, she mixed Clorox bleach with ammonia. She was then coughing and gagging.

1. What is the route of exposure?

2. How should the EMTs manage it?

CHAPTER 36
Prenatal Problems

An EMT may be called to the scene of a woman who is having a complication of pregnancy. He now has two lives to consider, but prompt attention to life-threatening complications can help to ensure survival of both mother and child in many cases.

True or False: Read each statement and decide if it is true or false. Write T or F on the line before each statement.

1. _____ A woman with abdominal pain should be suspected of having appendicitis.
2. _____ A pregnancy outside the uterus is called an ectopic pregnancy.
3. _____ Ectopic pregnancies pose the greatest risk to the mother at nine months.
4. _____ The location of the ectopic pregnancy poses little risk of hemorrhage or shock.
5. _____ Hypotension is normal during an ectopic pregnancy.
6. _____ Vaginal bleeding during pregnancy should be considered serious.
7. _____ Premature separation of the placenta from the uterus is called a prolapse.
8. _____ Placenta previa is when the placenta grows over the cervix.
9. _____ Spontaneous abortions are also called miscarriages.
10. _____ Seat belts decrease maternal and infant mortality.

Identification: Read each definition and write the correct word or phrase it describes.

1. ______________________ Loss of a pregnancy
2. ______________________ A convulsive disorder seen only in pregnancy
3. ______________________ The afterbirth grows over the cervix
4. ______________________ Compression of the vena cava with a drop in blood pressure when the pregnant woman lies flat
5. ______________________ An inflammation of the appendix
6. ______________________ Nonmedical term used to describe a loss of a pregnancy, usually early in the pregnancy
7. ______________________ A pregnancy outside the uterus
8. ______________________ The afterbirth prematurely dislodges from the uterine wall

Fill in the Blank: Complete each sentence by filling in the missing word or words.

Pregnancy changes the way the body takes care of itself. The pregnant woman's heart is normally ______________ than the nonpregnant woman's, and her blood pressure is usually_________________. The EMT should remember that the pregnant woman has manufactured approximately _____% more blood than usual, and so a significant blood loss can occur before there is a change in ____________ ______________.

The EMT must remember that in managing any trauma in pregnancy, she must concentrate on saving the ______________.

Short Answer: Read each question. Think about the information presented in your text, and then answer each question with one or two sentences.

1. In addition to vital signs, what assessments should the EMT use in determining shock in the pregnant patient? Why?

2. Name at least three mechanisms of injury that are likely to cause trauma to the pregnant woman and fetus.

3. Why are pregnant women at risk for these mechanisms of injury?

Critical Thinking: Read the following scenario and then answer the questions.

The dispatcher had sent Denise and Steve to the Cassidy home for a "pregnancy-related" problem. Upon their arrival, they found Mrs. Cassidy lying on the couch. She stated that she was eight months pregnant, with the baby due in four weeks. That morning, while ironing, there was some bleeding from the vagina. The bleeding had increased, and she then called her doctor and 9-1-1.

1. List the assessments that the EMTs must make at this point.

Mrs. Cassidy told Steve that she did not have any pain with this bleeding, had not noticed any contractions, and did not injure herself.

2. What is the likely cause of Mrs. Cassidy's bleeding?

3. How should Steve and Denise manage Mrs. Cassidy?

CHAPTER 37
Emergency Childbirth

Even though pregnancy is a common condition, childbirth rarely occurs in the field! Although EMTs do not often encounter this type of situation, they must familiarize themselves with and review the basic principles of childbirth.

Word Scramble: Unscramble the following words. Use the clues to help you.

1. Thinning of the cervix — mtffnaccee ____________________
2. Process in which the fetus is expelled from the uterus — rolba ____________________
3. Term to describe a woman who has had children — prsouaitlmu ____________________
4. Term to describe a woman in her first pregnancy — soruapiirmp ____________________
5. Appearance of the fetal head at the vagina — growncin ____________________
6. Total number of pregnancies — vidarga ____________________
7. Total number of live children born to a woman — raap ____________________
8. Movement of the cranial bones in a delivering fetus — gomlind ____________________
9. Fetal stool — nocmmuie ____________________

Definitions: Write the definitions of the following terms.

1. amniotic sac ____________________
2. cervical dilation ____________________
3. bloody show ____________________
4. Braxton Hicks contractions ____________________
5. cardinal movements of labor ____________________
6. prolapsed umbilical cord ____________________
7. breech presentation ____________________
8. premature delivery ____________________

Sorting: Determine whether the description is of the first, second, or third stage of labor. Write the description under the correct stage.

effacement

delivery of the infant

rupture of the amniotic sac

delivery of the placenta

full cervical dilation

infant's head pushing on rectum

crowning

gushing of blood, approximately 250–500 cc

First stage **Second stage** **Third stage**

Identification: Place a checkmark in front of the essential components of a predelivery history.

_____ Due date

_____ Blood pressure

_____ Any complications during the pregnancy

_____ Crowning

_____ Prenatal care

_____ Any fluids from the vagina

_____ Time when contractions started

_____ BSI

_____ Maternal weight

_____ How long each contraction lasts

_____ Gravida

_____ Parity

Sorting: Decide if the EMT should assist the mother to deliver in the field or begin transport to the hospital. Put each situation under the likely location.

primiparous, contractions 10 minutes apart

crowning

irregular contractions

multiparous, contractions 2 minutes apart

need to move bowels

increased vaginal pressure

need to push

primiparous, regular contractions, no observation of fetal head

Field delivery **Transport**

Listing: State the use for each component in the OB kit.

1. surgical scissors
2. clamps

3. bulb suction
4. towels
5. gauze sponges
6. BSI
7. blanket
8. plastic bag

Ordering: Place the following steps for a field delivery in order. Place a numeral 1 before the first step, a 2 before the second step, and so on.

_____ Deliver placenta

_____ Position the mother

_____ Gentle pressure on the infant's head during crowning

_____ Check for cord around the neck

_____ Record time and place of delivery

_____ Suction mouth and then nose of infant

_____ BSI

_____ Clamp cord when pulsations have stopped

_____ Dry infant and wrap

_____ Support the infant's weight during delivery

_____ Transport mother, infant, and placenta to hospital

Critical Thinking: Read the following scenario and then answer the questions.

Deb and Rhonda, both EMTs, arrived at the home of Grace Hayfield, a 22-year-old female. Grace was expecting her first child and believed that labor had begun. When Deb and Rhonda asked her due date, she told them the baby was not due for four weeks but she was having intense contractions every four minutes, and her water had broken. While Deb prepared to perform a discreet visual exam of the perineum, Rhonda asked about prenatal care. Grace confessed that she had never seen a doctor for the pregnancy because she did not have any insurance, and the baby's father was not willing to assist. Deb informed Rhonda that the infant's head was present at the vaginal opening, and delivery was imminent.

1. What equipment will Deb and Rhonda need for the field delivery?
2. What should the EMTs tell Grace regarding the plan of care?
3. Should the EMTs contact Medical Control? Why or why not?

The field delivery proceeded without a hitch—a beautiful baby girl who was breathing well on her own, crying loudly, and turning nice and pink. Deb said she would complete the newborn assessment while Rhonda prepared to deliver the placenta. Rhonda noted that Grace still appeared "very pregnant" and the placenta had not appeared.

4. What is the likely explanation for Grace's appearance?
5. What should the EMTs do now?

Chapter 37 Skill Sheet

Student Name ______________________________ Date ________________

Skill 37-1: Emergency Delivery

Equipment Needed:

1. Surgical scissors or cord clamps
2. Bulb suction device
3. Towels
4. Gauze sponges
5. Baby blanket
6. Sanitary napkins
7. Plastic bag or bucket
8. Personal protective equipment

Yes: ❑ Reteach: ❑ Return: ❑ Instructor initials: ________

Step 1: Position the mother supine, with knees drawn up and spread apart, and assist by helping her to elevate her buttocks on a pillow or blankets.

Yes: ❑ Reteach: ❑ Return: ❑ Instructor initials: ________

Step 2: Create a clean area around the vaginal opening with clean towels or paper barriers.

Yes: ❑ Reteach: ❑ Return: ❑ Instructor initials: ________

Step 3: As the infant's head appears during crowning, place fingers gently on the skull and exert very gentle pressure to prevent explosive delivery.

Yes: ❑ Reteach: ❑ Return: ❑ Instructor initials: ________

Step 4: If the amniotic sac has not broken, use thumb and forefinger, or a clamp, to puncture the sac and push it away from the infant's head and face.

Yes: ❑ Reteach: ❑ Return: ❑ Instructor initials: ________

Step 5: As the infant's head is delivered, determine if the umbilical cord is around the neck; if it is, slip it over the infant's head or shoulder. If it is not possible to slip the cord, clamp the cord in two places, cut the cord between the clamps, and unwrap the cord from the infant's neck.

Yes: ❑ Reteach: ❑ Return: ❑ Instructor initials: ________

(continues)

Chapter 37 Skill Sheet

Skill 37-1: *Continued*

Step 6: After the infant's head is born, support the head and suction the newborn's mouth and then the nose several times with the bulb suction device.

Yes: ❑ Reteach: ❑ Return: ❑ Instructor initials: ________

Step 7: As the torso and full body are born, support the infant with both hands. As the feet are born, grasp them firmly.

Yes: ❑ Reteach: ❑ Return: ❑ Instructor initials: ________

Step 8: After pulsations cease in the umbilical cord, clamp the cord in two places, with the closest clamp about four fingers' width away from the infant, and then cut the cord between the clamps.

Yes: ❑ Reteach: ❑ Return: ❑ Instructor initials: ________

Step 9: Then gently dry the infant with towels and wrap the infant in a warm blanket. Place the infant on its side, preferably with the head slightly lower than the trunk.

Yes: ❑ Reteach: ❑ Return: ❑ Instructor initials: ________

Step 10: Another EMT should monitor the infant and complete initial care of the newborn.

Yes: ❑ Reteach: ❑ Return: ❑ Instructor initials: ________

Step 11: Place a sterile sanitary napkin between the mother's legs and have her close her legs. Also, comfort the mother and monitor vital signs.

Yes: ❑ Reteach: ❑ Return: ❑ Instructor initials: ________

Step 12: While preparing the mother and infant for transport, watch for delivery of the placenta. When the placenta is delivered, wrap the placenta in a towel and place it in a plastic bag or container, transporting it to the hospital with the mother.

Yes: ❑ Reteach: ❑ Return: ❑ Instructor initials: ________

CHAPTER 38
Newborn Care

Although most deliveries are without complications, an infant is at high risk for potentially fatal problems in the first hour of life.

True or False: Read each statement and decide if it is true or false. Write T or F on the line before each statement.

1. _____ A newborn with hypoxia is usually tachycardic.
2. _____ Pad the shoulders to keep the infant's airway in neutral position.
3. _____ The EMT should suction the infant's airway for no longer than three seconds.
4. _____ The infant's tongue is smaller proportionally than the adult's.
5. _____ There is no exchange of drugs from mother to her unborn infant.
6. _____ Start chest compressions on a newborn with a heart rate below 60 beats per minute.
7. _____ The EMT should perform three compressions to each ventilation in infant CPR.
8. _____ Meconium is a white, cheesy material designed to protect the newborn.
9. _____ Acrocyanosis is a severe birth defect.
10. _____ The EMT can usually palpate only two fontanelles on the newborn.

Sorting: Place a checkmark in front of the circumstances that can lead to hypothermia in the newborn. Suggest a way to correct those circumstances.

1. _____ suckling
2. _____ placing the newborn on a table
3. _____ positioning the newborn on mother's abdomen
4. _____ leaving baby's head uncovered to monitor fontanelles
5. _____ letting infant stay in amniotic fluid
6. _____ swaddling

Ordering: Place the following management techniques into the correct order. Place a numeral 1 before the first thing to be done, a 2 before the next, and so on.

_____ ALS drugs

_____ Blow-by oxygen

_____ Chest compressions

_____ Drying, warming, and positioning

_____ BVM

Fill in the Blank: Complete each sentence by filling in the missing word or words.

Measuring heart rate, respiratory effort, muscle tone, responses, and color in the newborn is determined through the use of the __________________ score. It is completed at ____________, and ___________ minutes after birth. The EMT must also assess the newborn's airway. Place the newborn supine and slightly head down. Use a ____________ _____________ to clear the newborn's _________________. The newborn is an obligate ______________ breather. Respirations must be adequate. Crying is a good sign. Even though respirations are adequate, the infant may have blue hands and feet. This is called _________________________. A heart rate of less than ______ beats per minute means that the EMT must begin chest compressions. Once the initial assessment and Apgar is completed, begin a ____________________ medical assessment. Sometimes the newborn's head may appear misshapen. This results from the birth and is called __________________. The head shape will return to normal. The EMT must assess the __________________ cord, which should appear bluish white. The EMT must take care to appear professional and nonjudgmental, as new parents "read" the expressions and behaviors of the caregivers.

Calculation: Calculate the Apgar for each of the following newborns.

1. Newborn is crying loudly, kicking, heart rate of 120 beats per minute, sneezing after suctioning with pink body and blue extremities
2. Newborn is crying weakly, blue body and extremities, heart rate of 90, no reaction to suctioning, extended limbs
3. Newborn is crying weakly, blue body and extremities, heart rate of 110, sneezing, and clenching arms and legs to body
4. Newborn is not crying, body blue, limp extremities, heart rate of 80, no reaction to suction
5. Newborn has pink trunk and extremities, coughing with suction, heart rate of 135, legs and arms held in fetal position unless extended by EMT, crying loudly

Short Answer: Read each question. Think about the information presented in your text, and then answer each question with one or two sentences.

1. State at least two reasons why it is important to suction the newborn's nostrils.

2. List four indicators of respiratory distress in the newborn.

Critical Thinking: Read the following scenario and then answer the questions.

Donna and Jarrett, both EMTs, responded to a call for a woman in labor. Upon their arrival at the residence, they were met at the walk by Gary, an on-duty police officer who was also an EMT. Gary informed Jarrett, the crew chief, that Gary could not ride into the hospital on the ambulance, but that he could assist in any way that Jarrett needed. When they entered the residence, they found that Johanna, a 24-year-old mother of one, had delivered a tiny newborn in the bedroom. The newborn was apneic, bradycardic at 70 beats per minute, and cyanotic. He was not crying and did not seem to respond at all. Johanna was lying on the bed, crying. Her color was normal, her skin was warm and moist, with minimal bleeding from the vagina. The placenta had not yet delivered.

1. What is the newborn's Apgar?

2. Describe immediate care for the newborn.

3. What can the EMTs say to Johanna?

CHAPTER 39
Pediatric Medical Emergencies

Familiarity with techniques of pediatric assessment, and the common illnesses in each age group, can help the EMT to feel more comfortable when faced with an ill or injured child.

Word Scramble: Using the Key Terms in Chapter 39 of the textbook, unscramble the following.

1. upcor ______________________________
2. mathas ______________________________
3. inemgtnisi ______________________________
4. gettolitipis ______________________________
5. grebfinied ______________________________
6. noscittrcar ______________________________
7. relibef ______________________________

Completion: Complete the following table of developmental considerations and vital signs.

Age	Respiratory rate	Heart rate	Systolic blood pressure
Newborn			
6 weeks			
6 months			
1 year			
3 years			
6 years			
10 years			

True or False: Read each statement and decide if it is true or false. Place T or F on the line before each statement.

1. _____ Examine a painful extremity last.
2. _____ Newborns do not yet recognize their mothers.
3. _____ Never permit the mother to hold the infant during your exam.
4. _____ Infants usually double their birth weight by 5 months of age.
5. _____ The 8-month-old infant is usually afraid of strangers.
6. _____ A toe-to-head exam is less intimidating for the 10-month-old infant.
7. _____ Toddlers do not like to be separated from their parents.
8. _____ Ingestion of foreign bodies is a common problem for a newborn.
9. _____ Toddlers and preschoolers are at-risk for accidental burns.
10. _____ The EMT should always obtain a history from the parents, not the child.

11. ______ Body image is important to the teenaged patient.
12. ______ The greatest risk to a child with croup is a fever.
13. ______ The EMT should examine the mouth of a child who has a harsh, brassy cough.
14. ______ A simple cold can lead to difficulty breathing in a child.
15. ______ An increase in the respiratory rate is a sign of respiratory difficulty in a child.

Matching: Match each word or term with its definition.

1. ______ croup
2. ______ epiglottitis
3. ______ asthma
4. ______ SIDS
5. ______ meningitis
6. ______ febrile seizures
7. ______ dehydration
8. ______ diabetes
9. ______ gastroenteritis
10. ______ congenital disorder

a. present at birth
b. inflammation of the lining of the brain
c. results from rapid rise in temperature
d. lack of body water
e. marked by vomiting and diarrhea
f. bronchospasms and inflammation
g. unexplained death of an infant
h. bacterial infection with swelling
i. viral illness resulting in seal bark cough
j. Altered sugar metabolism

Correcting: The following statements are false. Replace the incorrect word or words and write the sentence as a true statement below.

1. The cause of SIDS is a <u>bacterial infection</u>.

2. SIDS rarely occurs in infants between the ages of <u>1 week and 6 months</u>.

3. SIDS usually occurs when the infant is <u>eating</u>.

4. <u>Larger</u> than normal birth weight babies are at increased risk for SIDS.

5. Full resuscitation is <u>not</u> done for SIDS.

6. SIDS <u>can</u> be prevented.

7. Parents can be informed of what was done for their child <u>at the hospital</u>.

8. EMTs caring for a SIDS child will <u>not</u> be stressed after the event.

Short Answer: Read each question. Think about the information presented in your text, and then answer each question with one or two sentences.

1. You are listening to the lungs of an otherwise healthy 2-year-old. She currently is having difficulty breathing. You hear air moving into the right lung, but not the left. Based on her age and her exam, what do think is the problem?

2. Both children and adults can develop the disease epiglottitis. Why is this disease more dangerous to a child than an adult?

3. Is it important for the EMT to differentiate croup from epiglottitis? Why or why not?

4. What are the signs of hypoperfusion in children?

Critical Thinking 1: Read the following scenario and then answer the questions.

Beth and Troy arrived at the Smythe home for a sick infant. Mrs. Smythe met them at the door, crying. She said her 16-month-old had a fever that morning. She gave her a dose of children's Tylenol, and placed her down for a nap. Now the infant was weak, listless, and not completely awake. There was also a rash over her upper body and shoulders.

1. Is there a potentially life-threatening condition present?

2. Based on the limited information available, what BSI should be taken?

3. What care do the EMTs need to provide to Mrs. Smythe?

Critical Thinking 2: Read the following scenario and then answer the questions.

Brent and Heidi responded to a call for a child "choking." Upon their arrival, they found a 6-year-old coughing vigorously. He was yelling that he never liked lima beans and that they made him choke.

1. Is there a potentially life-threatening condition present?

2. Based on the limited information available, what do Heidi and Brent know about the child's airway?

CHAPTER 40
Pediatric Trauma Emergencies

One of the most anxiety-producing emergencies for an EMT is pediatric trauma. Fortunately, the majority of pediatric trauma care involves integrating a few new facts into an already developed skill set. With practice, an EMT can become as comfortable with pediatric trauma as with adult trauma care.

Fill in the Blank: Read each of the following and then fill in the term it defines.

1. ____________________ Required by law to report suspicion of abuse
2. ____________________ A machine providing artificial breathing
3. ____________________ A catheter to drain excessive fluid from the brain
4. ____________________ Surgically created hole in neck extending to trachea
5. ____________________ Emotional, physical, or sexual harm to a child
6. ____________________ Flexible tube placed into stomach for nutrition
7. ____________________ Rigid tube placed in tracheostomy to maintain airway
8. ____________________ A special intravenous tube left in place for long periods

Identification: For each age group, list at least three likely mechanisms of injury.

Toddler ____

____

____

School-aged ____

____

____

Adolescent ____

____

____

Assessments: For each phase of the initial assessment, list at least two results that should concern the EMT regarding the status of the child.

General impression

Mental status

Airway

Breathing

Circulation

Short Answer: Read each question. Think about the information presented in your text, and then answer each question with one or two sentences.

1. A toddler and his mother tumble off a set of bleachers. Why is the toddler more likely to suffer a head injury?

2. Why would an EMT elect to keep a child in his car seat following a motor vehicle collision?

3. A toddler has been burned as the result of a small fire. In addition to burns, what other concerns should the EMT have regarding this child?

4. Give at least three examples of cases in which the EMT should consider child abuse. What should the EMT do if she does suspect abuse?

5. Why should the EMT caring for a child with special needs pay greater attention to caregiver information regarding vital signs and activities than her reference material?

Identification: Read each scenario and determine if the child should be transported to a level one trauma center or to a local hospital.

1. ______________________ A 3-year-old who fell from a 10-foot wall onto a paved driveway
2. ______________________ A 10-year-old with swollen, deformed, painful arm, with no punctures or lacerations from a skating injury
3. ______________________ A restrained 5-year-old in a low-speed, rear-end collision at the mall, seated mid-back seat
4. ______________________ A 6-year-old who was struck in head by a soccer ball, with immediate loss of consciousness
5. ______________________ A 12-year-old struck in face by a baseball, profuse bleeding from nose and mouth
6. ______________________ A 14-year-old fell off a snowmobile and was dragged through woods
7. ______________________ A 3-year-old with knife wound to thigh, sustained tachycardia
8. ______________________ An 11-year-old boy who cannot move after diving into shallow end of pool
9. ______________________ A 7-year-old with a 25 cent piece-sized burn from a flaming marshmallow
10. ______________________ An 8-year-old with tree branch impaled in back

CHAPTER 41
Geriatric Medical Emergencies

As our bodies age, there are characteristic changes that leave us susceptible to particular disease processes. Geriatrics is the study of the diseases of the older adult.

Matching: Match each word or term with its definition.

1. _____ arthritis
2. _____ delirium
3. _____ dementia
4. _____ elder abuse
5. _____ osteoporosis
6. _____ polypharmacy

a. acute change in level of consciousness
b. physical or emotional mistreatment of the elderly
c. progressive loss of calcium, weakening the bones
d. multiple medications by a single patient
e. gradual decline in intellectual and mental function
f. inflammation within the joints

Identification: For each system, list the common changes that occur as we age.

1. Visual
2. Hearing
3. Cardiovascular
4. Respiratory
5. Gastrointestinal
6. Genitourinary
7. Musculoskeletal
8. Integumentary

Fill in the Blank: Fill in the blanks regarding trauma and disease in the elderly.

In the over-65-years-old population, ________________ is the fifth leading cause of death. ________________ account for the most significant injuries in the adult. In obtaining a history, it is important for the EMT to question ________________ that occurred before any falls. Even minor ________________ trauma can lead to significant injury. Subtle symptoms such as ________________ or ________________ may occur days to weeks after the injury.

More than one half of all ________________ ________________ (MI) occur in elderly patients. Their symptoms may be unusual, including ________________ of ________________, ________________, ________________, ________________ or ________________ even without chest pain. Abdominal pain in an elderly patient can mean a ________________ ________________. Many elderly patients with severe infection do not have a ________________.

Many elderly patients suffer from ________________, which means the person may not be able to properly take care of himself. Additionally, ________________ abuse is common in the elderly population of the United States. ________________ can lead to immune compromise and resultant infections.

Short Answer: Read each question. Think about the information presented in your text, and then answer each question with one or two sentences.

1. What is the difference between delirium and dementia?

2. Why is it important for the EMT to make the distinction between the two conditions?

Critical Thinking: Read the following scenario and then answer the questions.

Martha Wittakers called 9-1-1. A strange elderly woman had arrived at her doorstep, claiming to live there. Mrs. Wittakers had tried to find where she lived but the woman was adamant that it was right here. When the EMTs, Tony and Lisa, arrived, Mrs. Wittakers was being served tea in her own kitchen by the elderly woman.

1. What is the likely cause of the elderly woman's situation?

2. Name other causes that the EMTs should consider.

While the EMTs were trying to gather any information from the elderly woman, their radio cackled. "Be on the alert for a 78-year-old female, wandered from an Adult Day Service area on Vine and Wisteria Street." Lisa advised the dispatchers of their current situation and requested a police unit to assist. Police arrived with the son of the missing woman.

3. Should the EMTs simply release the elderly woman to the son? Why or why not?

4. What should they do first?

5. What explanation should they give to the son?

6. Describe optimal care for the elderly woman.

CHAPTER 42
Advance Directives

Advances in medicine have made it possible to delay death. As we struggle with this, patients have begun to assert their rights to determine the course of their life and death.

Definitions: Write the definitions of the following terms.

1. advance directive ______________________________
2. DNR order ______________________________
3. health care proxy ______________________________
4. living will ______________________________
5. power of attorney ______________________________

True or False: Read each statement and decide if it is true or false. Write T or F on the line before each statement.

1. _____ Efforts to express the patient's wishes before he becomes incapacitated are called terminal directives.
2. _____ A person who is physically disabled cannot legally make end-of-life decisions.
3. _____ A disease in which there is no medical hope is called terminal.
4. _____ A durable power of attorney enables another person to make decisions for someone unable to make them.
5. _____ The Patient Self-Determination Act of 1991 protects the rights of patients and physicians.
6. _____ Hospice care provides care to patients only when hospitalized.
7. _____ Supportive care designed to ease a patient's suffering is called resuscitative care.
8. _____ An out-of-hospital DNR provides a medical order to EMTs.
9. _____ An agent, designated by a health care proxy or power of attorney, is someone entrusted to make decisions on behalf of the patient.
10. _____ Implied consent assumes that a patient would want treatment if he were able to express himself.

Short Answer: Read each question. Think about the information presented in your text, and then answer each question with one or two sentences.

1. What legal principles govern both withholding CPR and beginning CPR on an unconscious patient?

2. What are the differences between the living will and power of attorney versus a do not resuscitate (DNR) and health care proxy?

Critical Thinking 1: Read the following scenario and then answer the questions.

Bob and Greg were on their first call together. It came early, only a few minutes after the shift began. They received dispatch information for an unresponsive elderly woman. When the EMTs arrived at the house, they were met by the granddaughter. She handed them an out-of-hospital DNR signed by the patient's physician. Through her tears, she said her grandmother was adamant about not doing anything but she (the granddaughter) just was not certain her grandmother was dead.

1. What care is required for the grandmother at this point?

2. What care does the granddaughter need?

Critical Thinking 2: Read the following scenario and then answer the question.

Ambulance 4 responded to a large, old home in the northern section of town. The call was for an elderly man who had difficulty breathing. Upon their arrival, they found the man lying on the floor with several relatives around him. One young man was saying that a DNR order existed, but three other relatives yelled that the older man, their uncle, had changed his mind.

1. How should the EMTs respond to this situation?

CHAPTER 43
Emergency Vehicle Operations

In addition to the vast amount of medical knowledge that the new EMT will learn, he must also learn the basics of EMS operations.

Matching: Match each word or term with its definition.

1. _____ wave off
2. _____ panic stop
3. _____ rotor wash
4. _____ approach path
5. _____ landing zone
6. _____ flashback
7. _____ due regard
8. _____ shoreline
9. _____ sharps container
10. _____ right of way
11. _____ EVOC
12. _____ siren mode
13. _____ hot load
14. _____ spotter
15. _____ wigwags

a. area intended for the helicopter to come down
b. respect and consideration for others
c. privilege of moving ahead of others on a roadway
d. receptacle for used needles
e. emergency vehicle operators course
f. wind created by cycling of helicopter blades
g. placing a patient aboard a running helicopter
h. emergency stop for unexpected obstacle
i. alternating headlights on an emergency vehicle
j. a person who assists the driver in backing up
k. crossing and uncrossing of arms to alert pilot
l. obstacle-free area for helicopter to come in to land
m. electrical extension linking ambulance to building
n. strobes reflecting back into driver's eyes
o. characteristic patterns of sound alerting others to emergency

Definitions: Write the definitions of the following terms.

1. controlled intersection ______________________________
2. yelp ______________________________
3. LZ officer ______________________________
4. covering the brake ______________________________
5. surrounding area ______________________________
6. emergency ambulances ______________________________
7. four-second rule ______________________________
8. emergency services vehicle ______________________________
9. touchdown area ______________________________
10. wail ______________________________

Listing: List four considerations for personnel preparedness.

1. ______
2. ______
3. ______
4. ______

Listing: List six considerations for equipment readiness.

1. ______
2. ______
3. ______
4. ______
5. ______
6. ______

Listing: List at least 10 items for the vehicle safety checklist.

1. ______
2. ______
3. ______
4. ______
5. ______
6. ______
7. ______
8. ______
9. ______
10. ______

Listing: List at least eight items that should be placed in the vehicle front compartment.

1. ______
2. ______
3. ______
4. ______
5. ______
6. ______
7. ______
8. ______

Descriptions: Describe each phase of the call by giving an example of activities in each.

1. Alarm and alert

2. Initial information

3. Departure

4. Driving

5. Arrival

6. On-scene actions

7. Transport to facility

8. Arrival at facility

9. Transfer of care

10. Preparation for next call

Short Answer: Read the question. Think about the information presented in your text, and then answer the question with one or two sentences.

What is ƎƆИA⅃UᙠMA?

Critical Thinking 1: Read the following scenario and then answer the questions.

"Car versus train" was the dispatch. Janie and Brad, EMTs with Response Rescue, both thought this would be a bad one. Upon their arrival, they saw a freight train stopped on the tracks about 50 feet past the intersection of the roadway and the tracks. The remains of a blue car were at the front left side of the train. The driver of the car was trapped but alive. He was talking to the engineer. Janie gathered a history of events and called a report back to communications. Brad began the initial assessment. The train had been slow moving and had begun to brake almost two miles back. As such, it was close to stopping at the point of impact. For some unknown reason the driver had not left his car. Initial assessment revealed blunt injury to the chest and an open femur fracture; extrication would be lengthy. They decided to call for a helicopter to transport to the trauma center.

1. Do you agree with the decision to call the helicopter? Why or why not?

2. Describe how the LZ officer will assist in landing the helicopter.

Critical Thinking 2: Read the following scenario and then answer the questions.

Ericka and Katrina had just picked up dinner. Wow, they were actually going to eat by 5:30 P.M.! But the tones went out for a priority call on the other side of the city. Resigned, they put their raincoats back on and climbed into the rig.

1. What driving hazards are present as the EMTs answer this call?

2. How should the EMTs handle each hazard?

CHAPTER 44 Public Safety Incident Management

A response to a scene with multiple patients or unknown chemical exposures may be very stressful and confusing. It is the responsibility of the EMT to bring order to these situations.

Definitions: Write the definition of the following terms.

1. chain of command ____________________
2. command post ____________________
3. decontamination corridor ____________________
4. hot zone ____________________
5. material safety data sheets (MSDS) ____________________
6. multiple casualty incident (MCI) ____________________
7. NFPA 704 symbol ____________________
8. START triage system ____________________
9. placard ____________________
10. triage ____________________

Matching: Match each word or term with its definition.

1.	_____ incident command		a.	personnel to stop hazmat spillage
2.	_____ EMS command		b.	decides urgency of patient's illnesses
3.	_____ public safety officer		c.	has responsibility for an incident
4.	_____ research officer		d.	in charge of organizing care of patients
5.	_____ safety officer		e.	gathers information about hazmat
6.	_____ staging officer		f.	has responsibility for EMS at incident
7.	_____ transportation officer		g.	responsible for safety of all personnel
8.	_____ treatment officer		h.	organizes pre- and hospital resources
9.	_____ triage officer		i.	reports state of affairs to the media
10.	_____ operations level responder		j.	assembles and assigns duties to personnel

Identification: Assuming you have two ambulances on scene and another en route, mark each of the following as green, yellow, red, or black, according to the color triage tag you would assign.

1. ____________ A 28-year-old female with abdominal cramps, who states she is pregnant
2. ____________ A 34-year-old male limping, who says his right ankle hurts
3. ____________ A 46-year-old male with a respiratory rate of 36, who is desperately looking for his inhaler
4. ____________ A 20-year-old female with a painful and deformed left wrist
5. ____________ A 77-year-old male with chest pain on a 10 out of 10 pain scale, with good respirations and pulse
6. ____________ A 4-year-old female, who is still apneic, after a jaw thrust is initiated

7. ______________ A 16-year-old with an amputated right leg below the thigh and respirations of 24, who is without a radial pulse
8. ______________ A 58-year-old male with a weak radial pulse, who can only breathe if his airway is held open
9. ______________ A 36-year-old female with a possible dislocated shoulder, without a distal pulse
10. ______________ A 90-year-old female in cardiac arrest

Ordering: Place the following events in the order in which they should occur at an incident. Put a numeral 1 before the first action, a 2 before the next, and so on.

_____ Warm zone is established with a decontamination corridor

_____ Hot zone is established

_____ Hazmat team is dispatched

_____ The first unit arrives at the scene of a rolled over tanker truck

_____ Patients are extracted from the tanker

_____ Patients are decontaminated

_____ Patients are treated

_____ EMS command is established

_____ Patients are transported

_____ Ambulance is staged in the cold zone

Fill in the Blank: Fill in the blanks in the START triage algorithm.

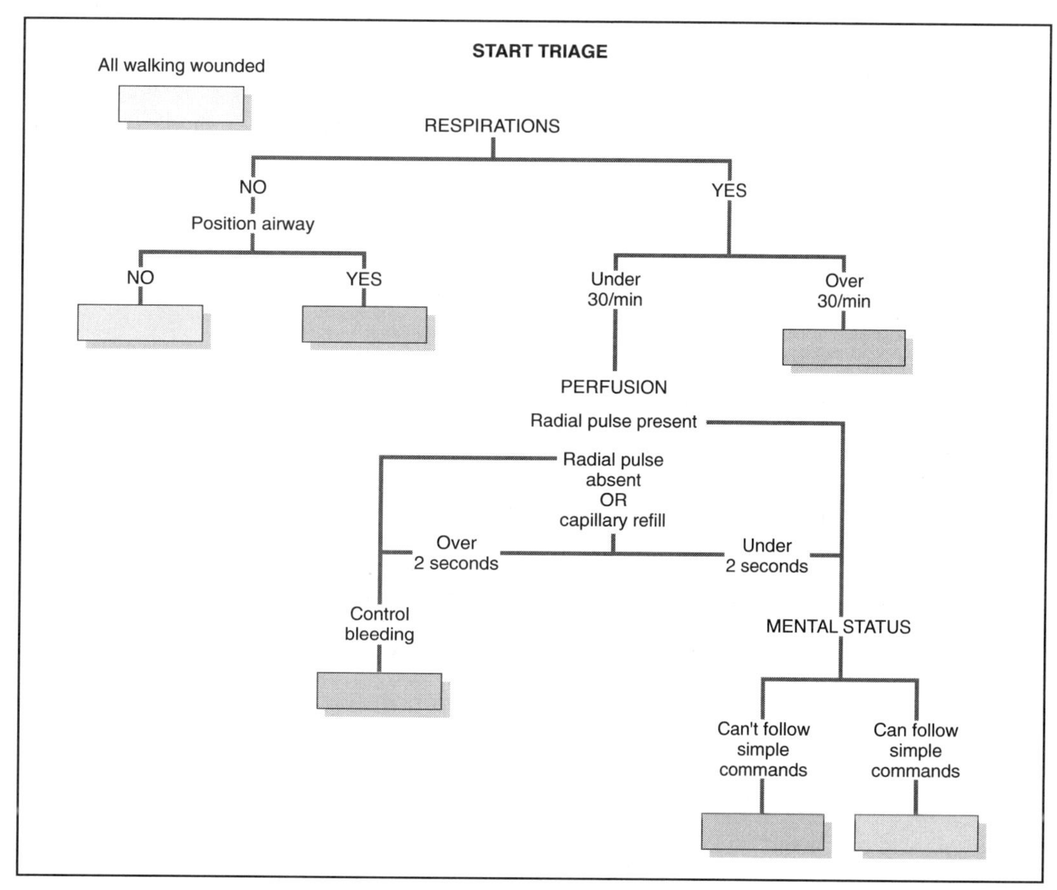

Research: Using the *Emergency Response Guidebook*, find the name of each substance.

1. placard 2717
2. placard 1203
3. placard 1046
4. placard 1680
5. placard 1274

Using the *Emergency Response Guidebook*, find the placard number of each substance.

6. lithium
7. zinc nitrate
8. strychnine
9. oxygen
10. copper chloride

Using the *Emergency Response Guidebook*, find the first aid requirements for exposure to the following.

11. placard 2902

Short Answer: Read the question. Think about the information presented in your text, and then answer the question with one or two sentences.

What does the mnemonic SIN stand for?

Critical Thinking 1: Read the following scenario and then answer the questions.

"Quality Ambulance Units 1, 2, and 3, respond to Highway 84 for reports of a tour bus off road. Multiple injuries. Time out 1600." Unit 2 arrived at scene first to find a full-sized tour bus overturned. Many people were milling about, and others were screaming or crying.

1. What is the role of Unit 2?
2. What sectors need assignment?
3. How can Unit 2 handle the arrival of the media (e.g., TV reporters)?

Critical Thinking 2: Read the following scenario and then answer the questions.

Jean and Stephen answered a call for a truck struck by construction debris. Upon their approach, Jean saw a large tanker next to some huge steel girders. She told Stephen to stop the rig so she could get a better look. "Uh oh," she said, "It's leaking!"

1. List three ways that Jean and Stephen can find out what is in the truck.
2. Once a Hazmat scene has been recognized, what must the first arriving units do?
3. List the zones and who may enter.

CHAPTER 45
Rescue Operations

A rescue is an attempt to help another person who is incapable of freeing herself from confinement or danger. In order for a rescue to take place, there must be a live patient.

Matching: Match each word or term with its definition.

1.	_____	confined space	a.	the front of the car is pulled away
2.	_____	cribbing	b.	stays in one piece after being broken
3.	_____	flat water	c.	powerful down-currents
4.	_____	loaded bumpers	d.	used to stabilize a vehicle's frame
5.	_____	PFD	e.	last line of swift water rescue
6.	_____	roll the dash	f.	area with limited openings for entry or exit
7.	_____	safety glass	g.	a body without current
8.	_____	snag lines	h.	personal flotation device
9.	_____	tempered glass	i.	hydraulic compression dangerous to EMS
10.	_____	undertow	j.	designed to shatter into tiny fragments

Identification: Identify each of the following as related to water rescue (W), vehicle rescue (V), or both (B).

1. _____ Forcible entry
2. _____ Cribbing
3. _____ Flapping of the roof
4. _____ Nader pin
5. _____ Point of contact
6. _____ Throw bag
7. _____ Window punch
8. _____ Undertow
9. _____ Swift current
10. _____ High life hazard

Identification: For each of the following situations, identify a safety item that rescuers should use.

1. Body fluids
2. Loud noises
3. Sharp objects
4. Flying debris
5. Poor visibility
6. Flash and flame
7. Falling objects

Short Answer: Read each question. Think about the information presented in your text, and then answer each question with one or two sentences.

1. Describe how a shore-based rescue is established for both swift and flat waters.

2. List the phases of a rescue.

3. What is the minimum personal protective equipment that an EMT should have when extricating a patient from a crashed motor vehicle?

Critical Thinking 1: Read the following scenario and then answer the questions.

A semi filled with sand blew out its front tire, careened across two lanes of traffic on the bridge, and came to rest on its side against the guard rails; the cab hung over the street below.

1. What type of rescue will be necessary?

2. List at least three safety hazards.

Critical Thinking 2: Read the following scenario and then answer the questions.

A rowing shell was struck by a motorized racing boat, approximately 15 feet from shore.

1. What type of rescue will be necessary?

2. List at least three safety hazards.

Critical Thinking 3: Read the following scenario and then answer the questions.

Three college friends explored a set of caves on private property. One of the students became trapped in a narrow shaft.

1. What type of rescue will be necessary?

2. List at least three safety hazards.

CHAPTER 46 Emergency Response to Terrorism

EMS, an integral part of the emergency response team, shares responsibility for crisis management and will be called on to respond to a terrorist incident.

True or False: Read each statement and decide if it is true or false. Place T or F on the line before each statement.

1. _____ Domestic terrorists are citizens of any nation who commit terrorist acts in the United States.
2. _____ Good safety precautions always involve complicated procedures.
3. _____ Awareness level responders participate in decontamination.
4. _____ Weapons of mass destruction were originally created to kill an entire population of a country.
5. _____ A dirty bomb is called a nuclear dispersion device.
6. _____ A Geiger counter should be worn by individual EMTs to measure radiation.
7. _____ Radiation pagers measure an EMT's exposure level so that care can be instituted.
8. _____ Biologic agents are bacterial, viral, and toxic.
9. _____ Chemical weapons can be divided into three classes.
10. _____ Secondary devices are designed to injure emergency response units.

Identification: List the agency responsible for each emergency support function.

1. Transportation ____________________
2. Communications ____________________
3. Public Works ____________________
4. Firefighting ____________________
5. Information/Planning ____________________
6. Mass Care ____________________
7. Resource Support ____________________
8. Health and Medical Services ____________________
9. Urban Search and Rescue ____________________
10. Hazardous Materials ____________________
11. Food ____________________
12. Energy ____________________

Matching: Place the letter of the correct example on the line in front of the element.

1. ____ L	a.	cold zone
2. ____ A	b.	portable radio
3. ____ C	c.	avoid blocking in vehicle
4. ____ E	d.	safety officer
5. ____ S	e.	minimum level of training

Short answer: List at least one way the EMT can prepare for each hazard in the mnemonic TRACEM.

1. T
2. R
3. A
4. C
5. E
6. M

Critical Thinking: Read the following case study and then answer the questions.

Corey and Tom were the first EMTs on the scene of a gas line rupture. The incident had occurred at the meeting rooms of a political group that was not well liked in this region. The regular planning meeting had been going on, so Corey knew there would be at least 15 people inside.

1. Is this a terrorist incident? Why or why not?
2. Name at least three hazards that may be present on this scene.
3. Should Corey and Tom approach the scene? Why or why not?

Fire officials determined that this incident was not simply a gas line rupture. There was evidence of radiation present and blasting caps and some wire.

4. What is the difference between irradiation and contamination?
5. What three ways exist to limit exposure to a radiation source?

CHAPTER 47
EMS in Rural America

Historically, farming has been one of America's most dangerous occupations. When EMS is called to a farm, it is likely that a true emergency exists and that providers will find special circumstances, unique to farming, present.

Missing Letters: Complete the puzzle using terms found in Chapter 47 of the textbook.

f _ _ _ chem _ _ _ _ _

_ _ a _ _ b _ _ _

tractor r _ _ _ _ _ _ _

_ _ _ _ _ _ m

_ e _ _ _

_ _ _ _ m _ _ _ _

_ _ e

operator _ _ r _ _

_ _ g _ _

_ _ _ _ e _ _

n _ _ _ _ _ _ _ dioxide

c _ _ _

_ _ _ i _ _ circle

_ _ _ _ _ e storage

_ _ _ s _ _

Definitions: Write the definitions of the following terms.

1. rollover protective structures ____________________
2. power takeoff ____________________
3. silo ____________________
4. silage ____________________
5. toxic organic dust syndrome ____________________

Completion: Complete the missing word or words in each sentence.

1. Three quarters of the United States is considered ________________.
2. The majority of injuries that occur on farms are during the months of __________, __________, and __________.
3. Most farm emergencies are ________________ in nature.
4. EMTs should approach scenes cautiously and look for possible __________ __________.
5. When encountering heavy farm equipment, the EMT should call for __________ __________.

6. The EMT should ______________ his ________________ after encounters with farm animals.
7. To avoid being kicked by a horse, the EMT should walk____________ the animal.
8. The majority of farm injuries are due to ___________________ _____________.

Identification: Spell out each letter of the mnemonic SLUDGEM, referring to Table 46-2 in Chapter 46 of the textbook, then answer the questions.

S

L

U

D

G

E

M

1. In what way does SLUDGEM apply to farm incidents?

2. What is the treatment for this type of incident?

Short Answer: Read each question. Think about the information presented in your text, and then answer each question with one or two sentences.

1. List the three likely mechanisms of action in farm incidents.

2. List at least five special equipment/procedures for farm rescues.

Critical Thinking: Read the following case study and then answer the questions.

Jamie and Gerard were called to the Schoonmaker farm for a man down. No further information was yet available. Upon their arrival, Jessie Schoonmaker met them, crying that her father, Leo, had collapsed in the silo. It was just filled during the past two weeks and he was checking on packed silage.

1. What hazards exist for Jamie and Gerard?

2. What clues may exist regarding oxygen conditions at the silo?

3. Should Jamie and Gerard attempt to rescue Mr. Schoonmaker? Why or why not?

4. Describe an appropriate plan for this incident.

APPENDIX A
Advanced Airway Control

For a patient in need of extended airway maintenance, more secure means of stabilization may be required.

Definitions: Write the definitions of the following terms. Then state the indications for each.

1. Capnography ____
2. Pulse oximetry ____
3. Dual lumen airway device ____
4. Laryngeal mask airway ____

Identification: Place a checkmark in front of each patient requiring endotracheal intubation by the trained EMT-B.

_____ An unconscious patient in respiratory distress with an OPA in place

_____ A patient who states that it hurts to breathe

_____ A pulseless and apneic patient

_____ An unresponsive patient who has taken an overdose of narcotics

_____ A seizing patient with a paramedic expected to arrive in five minutes

_____ A patient who is choking on meat but is coughing forcefully

_____ A patient with facial injuries who has gagged on an OPA

_____ Driver in a car versus tree collision; CPR in progress

Matching: Match each word or term with its definition.

1. ____ gloves, mask, eye protection	a.	straight laryngoscope blade
2. ____ orogastric tube	b.	plastic tube placed in nose to stomach
3. ____ end tidal CO_2 detector	c.	opening on side of distal end of ET tube
4. ____ oxygen tank	d.	rigid guide placed in ET tube
5. ____ nasogastric tube	e.	curved laryngoscope blade
6. ____ laryngoscope handle	f.	plastic tube placed in mouth to stomach
7. ____ Macintosh blade	g.	plastic tube placed in the trachea
8. ____ Miller blade	h.	holds the batteries for direct laryngoscopy
9. ____ ET tube	i.	inserts air into cuff
10. ____ stylet	j.	maintains seal when inflated
11. ____ syringe	k.	helps prevent infection
12. ____ OPA	l.	holds medicinal gas
13. ____ cuff	m.	indicates pressure of carbon dioxide
14. ____ Murphy eye	n.	may be used as a bite block

Definitions: Write the definitions of the following terms.

1. pneumothorax ______________________
2. hyperventilate ______________________
3. aspiration ______________________
4. tension pneumothorax ______________________
5. direct laryngoscopy ______________________
6. endotracheal intubation ______________________

True or False: Read each statement and decide if it is true or false. Place T or F on the line before each statement.

1. _____ The vallecula is tissue covering the larynx.
2. _____ A cartilaginous flap of tissue at the base of the tongue is the epiglottis.
3. _____ The trachea connects the bronchii and the larynx.
4. _____ The upper jaw is the mandible.
5. _____ The opening at the vocal cords is the narrowest part of a child's airway.
6. _____ Cricoid pressure closes the epiglottis.
7. _____ The cricoid ring is the narrowest part of an adult's airway.
8. _____ Sniffing position is when the head is pushed forward toward the chest.
9. _____ The tongue must be moved to the right side of the mouth for endotracheal intubation.
10. _____ The carina is the point of bifurcation of the mainstem bronchii.

Ordering: Place the following actions in the order in which they should be performed for endotracheal intubation. Put a numeral 1 before the first action, a 2 before the next, and so on.

_____ Assess patient

_____ Lift blade upward and visualize the cords

_____ Ventilate and confirm placement

_____ Place distal end of tube through the opening between the cords

_____ Secure tube and reassess patient

_____ Assemble and test equipment

_____ Place OPA and hyperventilate the patient

_____ Remove blade

_____ Place blade into right side of patient's mouth and sweep the tongue left

_____ Lubricate and place stylet

_____ Place patient in sniffing position (provided there is no trauma)

_____ Stop ventilation

_____ Instill air into the pilot balloon and remove syringe

Short Answer: Describe how each method of tube placement confirmation works.

1. Visualization

2. Auscultation

3. Aspirator

4. CO_2 detector

5. Patient assessment

Short Answer: Describe how to correct each of the following situations during or after intubation.

1. What do the letters "DOPE" stand for in relation to ETT?

2. Upon auscultation, air movement is detected over the stomach. There is no chest rise.

3. The pilot balloon will not hold air and the patient can make sounds around the tube.

4. The stylet protrudes beyond the Murphy eye.

5. There are good breath sounds over the right lung but none over the left lung.

Critical Thinking 1: Read the following case study and then answer the questions.

Luke, Maria, and Chris were called to the home of Mr. King, a middle-aged man with a history of respiratory difficulties. While assessing the patient and setting up equipment, Mr. King stopped breathing.

1. What should the EMTs do?

While Maria and Chris were completing the BLS tasks, Luke contacted their dispatcher. A paramedic unit was dispatched to the scene and would arrive in 3–5 minutes.

2. What should Maria and Chris do now?

3. What information should be given to the paramedics upon their arrival?

4. What equipment should be ready for the paramedics?

Critical Thinking 2: Read the following case study and then answer the questions.

Denise and Steve were just completing a standby at the ski center located 45 minutes from the nearest hospital, when they were sent to a skier versus tree. The young man had struck the tree at a high rate of speed and was lying supine on the snowy slope. Bystanders had taken C-spine stabilization and were waiting for the EMTs. The young man was making snoring and gurgling noises.

1. What should Denise and Steve do now?

While continuing their assessment, the young man stopped breathing.

2. How should Denise and Steve manage the young man's airway?

3. Describe the process they should use to properly manage it.

Appendix A Skill Sheet

Student Name ______________________________ Date ________________

Skill A-1: Assembly of Laryngoscope and Blade

Equipment Needed:

1. Appropriate PPE
2. Laryngoscope handle
3. Variety of blade types and sizes
4. Spare lightbulbs and batteries

Yes: ❑ Reteach: ❑ Return: ❑ Instructor initials: ________

Step 1: The proximal end of the blade has a notched end that fits onto the handle securely.

Yes: ❑ Reteach: ❑ Return: ❑ Instructor initials: ________

Step 2: The notched end of the blade should be firmly attached to the handle with the blade in a closed position.

Yes: ❑ Reteach: ❑ Return: ❑ Instructor initials: ________

Step 3: Once properly attached, the blade can be extended, and the lightbulb at its distal end should turn on. The bulb should quickly be checked for security in position (be sure it is tightly screwed on), and bright quality of light. If the light is dim, the bulb may be poorly connected or the batteries may be low. It is the EMT's responsibility at the beginning of a shift to check the handles and blades to be sure they are functioning optimally.

Yes: ❑ Reteach: ❑ Return: ❑ Instructor initials: ________

Appendix A Skill Sheet

Student Name ______________________________ Date ________________

Skill A-2: Oral Endotracheal Intubation

Equipment Needed:

1. Laryngoscope
2. Endotracheal tubes (assorted)
3. Plastic-covered stylet
4. Water-soluble lubricant
5. Syringe (10 cc-minimum)
6. One-inch tape
7. Padding
8. Stethoscope
9. End tidal CO_2 detector

Yes: ❑ Reteach: ❑ Return: ❑ Instructor initials: ________

Step 1: Open, assess, suction, and secure the patient's airway with an oral airway. Ventilate the patient for 1–2 minutes.

Yes: ❑ Reteach: ❑ Return: ❑ Instructor initials: ________

Step 2: Assemble and prepare the intubation equipment. A correctly sized endotracheal tube should be chosen and the cuff tested, while the tube is in the packaging.

Yes: ❑ Reteach: ❑ Return: ❑ Instructor initials: ________

Step 3: The EMT then lubricates the stylet and inserts it into the endotracheal tube, stopping before the Murphy eye at the end of the tube. The entire assembly should be bent into a hockey-stick configuration.

Yes: ❑ Reteach: ❑ Return: ❑ Instructor initials: ________

Step 4: The EMT then assembles the laryngoscope handle and blade, ensuring that the bulb is "bright and tight."

Yes: ❑ Reteach: ❑ Return: ❑ Instructor initials: ________

Step 5: After positioning the patient's head in the sniffing position, by placing a 1½-inch pad under the head, the EMT directs another EMT to provide cricoid pressure.

Yes: ❑ Reteach: ❑ Return: ❑ Instructor initials: ________

Step 6: The first EMT stops ventilation and quickly removes the oral airway, inserting the blade, with his left hand, into the right side of the mouth and sweeping the tongue to the left and out of the way.

Yes: ❑ Reteach: ❑ Return: ❑ Instructor initials: ________

(continues)

Appendix A Skill Sheet

Skill A-2: *Continued*

Step 7: The EMT then identifies the landmarks of the airway. The vocal cords should be clearly visible, and the glottic opening identified.

Yes: ❑ Reteach: ❑ Return: ❑ Instructor initials: ________

Step 8: Without losing sight of the glottic opening, and while maintaining the up-and-out pressure on the laryngoscope blade, the EMT watches the tube pass through the glottic opening.

Yes: ❑ Reteach: ❑ Return: ❑ Instructor initials: ________

Step 9: Once the tube is in place, the EMT quickly withdraws the blade and the stylet, then inflates the balloon with the syringe.

Yes: ❑ Reteach: ❑ Return: ❑ Instructor initials: ________

Step 10: After inflating the balloon, the EMT removes the syringe and prepares to listen for lung sounds. First, the EMT must have another EMT place the BVM on the tube and begin ventilation. The EMT should never let go of the endotracheal tube until it has been secured.

Yes: ❑ Reteach: ❑ Return: ❑ Instructor initials: ________

Step 11: Using a stethoscope, the EMT first listens for the absence of sounds in the epigastric area, then proceeds to listen to lung sounds in the left lung, then the right lung.

Yes: ❑ Reteach: ❑ Return: ❑ Instructor initials: ________

Step 12: Using an end tidal CO_2 detector, the EMT confirms tube placement while also observing the torso for even chest rise.

Yes: ❑ Reteach: ❑ Return: ❑ Instructor initials: ________

Step 13: If the tube is misplaced, the syringe should be reattached, the balloon deflated, and the tube removed while suction is ready at the standby.

Yes: ❑ Reteach: ❑ Return: ❑ Instructor initials: ________

Step 14: If the tube is well placed, then the EMT proceeds to secure the tube with 1-inch tape or some similar securing device for that purpose.

Yes: ❑ Reteach: ❑ Return: ❑ Instructor initials: ________

NREMT Skill Sheet

Ventilatory Management: Endotracheal Intubation

Start Time: ________ **Stop Time:** ________ **Date:** ________________

Candidate's Name: ______________________________

Evaluator's Name: ______________________________

Note: *If a candidate elects to initially ventilate the patient with a BVM attached to a reservoir and oxygen, full credit must be awarded for steps denoted by "**" provided the first ventilation is delivered within the initial 30 seconds*		Points Possible	Points Awarded
Takes or verbalizes body substance isolation precautions		1	
Opens the airway manually		1	
Elevates the patient's tongue and inserts a simple airway adjunct (oropharyngeal/nasopharyngeal airway)		1	
Note: The examiner must now inform the candidate "no gag reflex is present and the patient accepts the airway adjunct."			
** Ventilates the patient immediately using a BVM device unattached to oxygen		1	
** Hyperventilates the patient with room air		1	
Note: The examiner must now inform the candidate that ventilation is being properly performed without difficulty.			
Attaches the oxygen reservoir to the BVM		1	
Attaches the BVM to high flow oxygen (15 liters per minute)		1	
Ventilates the patient at the proper volume and rate (800–1200 ml/breath and 10–20 breaths/minute)		1	
Note: After 30 seconds, the examiner must auscultate the patient's chest and inform the candidate that breath sounds are present and equal bilaterally and medical direction has ordered endotracheal intubation. The examiner must now take over ventilation of the patient.			
Directs assistant to hyper-oxygenate the patient		1	
Identifies/selects the proper equipment for endotracheal intubation		1	
Checks equipment	Checks for cuff leaks	1	
	Checks laryngoscope operation and bulb tightness	1	
Note: The examiner must remove the OPA and move out of the way when the candidate is prepared to intubate the patient.			
Positions the patient's head properly		1	
Inserts the laryngoscope blade into the patient's mouth while displacing the patient's tongue laterally		1	
Elevates the patient's mandible with the laryngoscope		1	
Introduces the endotracheal tube and advances the tube to the proper depth		1	
Inflates the cuff to the proper pressure		1	
Disconnects the syringe from the cuff inlet port		1	
Directs assistant to ventilate the patient		1	
Confirms proper placement of the endotracheal tube by auscultation bilaterally and over the epigastrium		1	
Note: The examiner must ask, "If you had proper placement, what would you expect to hear?"			
Secures the endotracheal tube *(may be verbalized)*		1	
	Total:	21	

Critical Criteria

_____ Did not take or verbalize body substance isolation precautions when necessary
_____ Did not initiate ventilation within 30 seconds after applying gloves or interrupts ventilation for greater than 30 seconds at any time
_____ Did not voice or provide high oxygen concentrations (15 liters/minute or greater)
_____ Did not ventilate the patient at a rate of at least 10 breaths per minute
_____ Did not provide adequate volume per breath (maximum of 2 errors per minute permissible)
_____ Did not hyper-oxygenate the patient prior to intubation
_____ Did not successfully intubate the patient within 3 attempts
_____ Used the patient's teeth as a fulcrum
_____ Did not assure proper tube placement by auscultation bilaterally over each lung and over the epigastrium
_____ The stylette (if used) extended beyond the end of the endotracheal tube
_____ Inserted any adjunct in a manner that was dangerous to the patient
_____ Did not immediately disconnect the syringe from the inlet port after inflating the cuff

NREMT Skill Sheet

Ventilatory Management: Dual Lumen Device Insertion Following an Unsuccessful Endotracheal Intubation Attempt

Start Time: ____________

Stop Time: ____________ **Date:** ________________

Candidate's Name: ______________________________

Evaluator's Name: ______________________________

		Points Possible	Points Awarded
Continues body substance isolation precautions		1	
Confirms the patient is being properly ventilated with high percentage oxygen		1	
Directs the assistant to hyper-oxygenate the patient		1	
Checks/prepares the airway device		1	
Lubricates the distal tip of the device *(may be verbalized)*		1	
Note: The examiner should remove the OPA and move out of the way when the candidate is prepared to insert the device.			
Positions the patient's head properly		1	
Performs a tongue-jaw lift		1	
❑ USES COMBITUBE	❑ USES THE PTL		
Inserts device in the mid-line and to the depth so that the printed ring is at the level of the teeth	Inserts the device in the mid-line until the bite blocks flange is at the level of the teeth	1	
Inflates the pharyngeal cuff with the proper volume and removes the syringe	Secures the strap	1	
Inflates the distal cuff with the proper volume and removes the syringe	Blows into tube #1 to adequately inflate both cuffs	1	
Attaches/directs attachment of BVM to the first (esophageal placement) lumen and ventilates		1	
Confirms placement and ventilation through the correct lumen by observing chest rise, auscultation over the epigastrium and bilaterally over each lung		1	
Note: The examiner states, "You do not see rise and fall of the chest and hear sounds only over the epigastrium."			
Attaches/directs attachment of BVM to the second (endotracheal placement) lumen and ventilates		1	
Confirms placement and ventilation through the correct lumen by observing chest rise, auscultation over the epigastrium and bilaterally over each lung		1	
Note: The examiner states, "You see rise and fall of the chest, there are no sounds over the epigastrium and breath sounds are equal over each lung."			
Secures device or confirms that the device remains properly secured		1	
	Total:	15	

Critical Criteria

_____ Did not take or verbalize body substance isolation precautions
_____ Did not initiate ventilation within 30 seconds
_____ Interrupted ventilations for more than 30 seconds at any time
_____ Did not hyper-oxygenate the patient prior to placement of the dual lumen airway device
_____ Did not provide adequate volume per breath (maximum of 2 errors/minute permissible)
_____ Did not ventilate the patient at a rate of at least 10 breaths per minute
_____ Did not insert the dual lumen airway device at a proper depth or at the proper place within 3 attempts
_____ Did not inflate both cuffs properly
_____ **Combitube** – Did not remove the syringe immediately following the inflation of each cuff
_____ **PTL** – Did not secure the strap prior to cuff inflation
_____ Did not confirm, by observing chest rise and auscultation over the epigastrium and bilaterally over each lung, that the proper lumen of the device was being used to ventilate the patient
_____ Inserted any adjunct in a manner that was dangerous to the patient

(Reprinted with permission of the National Registry of Emergency Medical Technicians.)

NREMT Skill Sheet

Ventilatory Management: Esophageal Obturator Airway Insertion Following an Unsuccessful Endotracheal Intubation Attempt

Start Time: ____________________

Stop Time: ____________________ **Date:** ______________

Candidate's Name: ____________________

Evaluator's Name: ____________________

	Points Possible	Points Awarded
Continues body substance isolation precautions	1	
Confirms the patient is being ventilated high percentage oxygen	1	
Directs the assistant to hyper-oxygenate the patient	1	
Identifies/selects the proper equipment for insertion of EOA	1	
Assembles the EOA	1	
Tests the cuff for leaks	1	
Inflates the mask	1	
Lubricates the tube *(may be verbalized)*	1	
Note: The examiner should remove the OPA and move out of the way when the candidate is prepared to insert the device.		
Positions the head properly with the neck in the neutral or slightly flexed position	1	
Grasps and elevates the patient's tongue and mandible	1	
Inserts the tube in the same direction as the curvature of the pharynx	1	
Advances the tube until the mask is sealed against the patient's face	1	
Ventilates the patient while maintaining a tight mask-to-face seal	1	
Directs confirmation of placement of EOA by obsserving for chest rise and auscultation over the epigastrium and bilaterally over each lung	1	
Note: The examiner must acknowledge adequate chest rise, bilateral breath sounds and absent sounds over the epigastrium.		
Inflates the cuff to the proper pressure	1	
Disconnects the syringe from the inlet port	1	
Continues ventilation of the patient	1	
Total:	17	

Critical Criteria

_______ Did not take or verbalize body substance isolation precautions
_______ Did not initiate ventilations within 30 seconds
_______ Interrupted ventilations for more than 30 seconds at any time
_______ Did not direct hyper-oxygenation of the patient prior to placement of the EOA
_______ Did not successfully place the EOA within 3 attempts
_______ Did not ventilate at a rate of at least 10 breaths per minute
_______ Did not provide adequate volume per breath (maximum 2 errors/minute permissible)
_______ Did not assure proper tube placement by auscultation bilaterally and over the epigastrium
_______ Did not remove the syringe after inflating the cuff
_______ Did not successfully ventilate the patient
_______ Did not provide high flow oxygen (15 liters per minute or greater)
_______ Inserted any adjunct in a manner that was dangerous to the patient

APPENDIX B Cardiopulmonary Resuscitation

CPR is performed to maintain circulation to the brain and heart until it can be shocked, that is, defibrillated, back into a normal rhythm.

Definitions: Write the definitions of the following terms.

1. sudden cardiac death ______________________________
2. look, listen, feel ______________________________
3. Heimlich maneuver ______________________________
4. advanced lividity ______________________________
5. return of spontaneous circulation ______________________________
6. rigor mortis ______________________________
7. signs of circulation ______________________________
8. quick check ______________________________

Short Answer: Read each question. Think about the information presented in your text, and then answer each question with one or two sentences.

1. List at least three circumstances in which CPR is performed as an assist to other treatments.

2. Name at least three situations in which the EMT would not start CPR.

3. How would the EMT check for responsiveness?

4. How would the EMT open the airway?

5. What is the EMT "looking, listening, and feeling" for?

6. Where is the carotid artery located?

7. Name at least three anatomical differences between children and adults that make CPR different for each.

Critical Thinking: Read the following scenario and then answer the questions.

Deborah and Steve responded to a "man down" call outside the local supermarket. When they arrived, they saw a middle-aged man lying supine on the ground with a citizen performing CPR. There was a crowd of people standing around and the parking lot was full.

1. What equipment should Steve bring to the patient's side?

2. Name at least four scene safety hazards involved with this call.

3. What are the differences between layperson CPR and EMR CPR?

4. How should Deborah and Steve proceed in continuing care for this patient?

Appendix B Skill Sheet

Student Name ______________________ Date __________

Foreign Body Airway Obstruction—Conscious Adult

Step 1: Ask if the person is choking.

Yes: ❑ Reteach: ❑ Return: ❑ Instructor initials: ________

Step 2: Perform the Heimlich maneuver or chest thrusts.

Yes: ❑ Reteach: ❑ Return: ❑ Instructor initials: ________

Step 3: Repeat until the obstruction is released.

Yes: ❑ Reteach: ❑ Return: ❑ Instructor initials: ________

If the person becomes unconscious:

Step 4: Call for advanced assistance.

Yes: ❑ Reteach: ❑ Return: ❑ Instructor initials: ________

Step 5: Open the airway with a tongue/jaw lift and finger sweep.

Yes: ❑ Reteach: ❑ Return: ❑ Instructor initials: ________

Step 6: Keeping the airway open, try to ventilate.

Yes: ❑ Reteach: ❑ Return: ❑ Instructor initials: ________

Step 7: If unable to ventilate, perform five abdominal thrusts or chest thrusts.

Yes: ❑ Reteach: ❑ Return: ❑ Instructor initials: ________

Step 8: Repeat steps 5, 6 and 7.

Yes: ❑ Reteach: ❑ Return: ❑ Instructor initials: ________

Appendix B Skill Sheet

Student Name ______________________ Date ____________

Foreign Body Airway Obstruction—Conscious Child

Step 1: Ask if the person is choking.

Yes: ❑ Reteach: ❑ Return: ❑ Instructor initials: ________

Step 2: Perform the Heimlich maneuver or chest thrusts.

Yes: ❑ Reteach: ❑ Return: ❑ Instructor initials: ________

Step 3: Repeat until the obstruction is released.

Yes: ❑ Reteach: ❑ Return: ❑ Instructor initials: ________

If the person becomes unconscious:

Step 4: Call for advanced assistance.

Yes: ❑ Reteach: ❑ Return: ❑ Instructor initials: ________

Step 5: Open the airway with a tongue/jaw lift and remove the object if you can see it.

Yes: ❑ Reteach: ❑ Return: ❑ Instructor initials: ________

Step 6: Keeping the airway open, try to ventilate.

Yes: ❑ Reteach: ❑ Return: ❑ Instructor initials: ________

Step 7: If unable to ventilate, perform five abdominal thrusts or chest thrusts.

Yes: ❑ Reteach: ❑ Return: ❑ Instructor initials: ________

Step 8: Repeat steps 5, 6 and 7.

Yes: ❑ Reteach: ❑ Return: ❑ Instructor initials: ________

Appendix B Skill Sheet

Student Name ______________________________ Date ________________

Foreign Body Airway Obstruction—Conscious Infant

Step 1: Check for breathing difficulty, ineffective cough, and absent or weak cry.

Yes: ❑ Reteach: ❑ Return: ❑ Instructor initials: ________

Step 2: Give five back blows and five chest thrusts until the obstruction is relieved.

Yes: ❑ Reteach: ❑ Return: ❑ Instructor initials: ________

If the infant becomes unconscious:

Step 3: Call for advanced assistance.

Yes: ❑ Reteach: ❑ Return: ❑ Instructor initials: ________

Step 4: Open the airway with a tongue/jaw lift and remove the object if you can see it.

Yes: ❑ Reteach: ❑ Return: ❑ Instructor initials: ________

Step 5: Keeping the airway open, try to ventilate.

Yes: ❑ Reteach: ❑ Return: ❑ Instructor initials: ________

Step 6: If unable to ventilate, perform five back blows and chest thrusts.

Yes: ❑ Reteach: ❑ Return: ❑ Instructor initials: ________

Step 7: Repeat steps 4, 5 and 6.

Yes: ❑ Reteach: ❑ Return: ❑ Instructor initials: ________

Appendix B Skill Sheet

Student Name ______________________ Date ____________

CPR for Adults—One or Two Rescuers

Step 1: Establish unresponsiveness.

Yes: ❑ Reteach: ❑ Return: ❑ Instructor initials: ________

Step 2: Have the second person obtain an AED or call for advanced assistance.

Yes: ❑ Reteach: ❑ Return: ❑ Instructor initials: ________

Step 3: Open the airway.

Yes: ❑ Reteach: ❑ Return: ❑ Instructor initials: ________

Step 4: Look, listen, and feel.

Yes: ❑ Reteach: ❑ Return: ❑ Instructor initials: ________

Step 5: If there is no breathing, give two slow breaths. (Suction the airway before ventilations, if needed.)

Yes: ❑ Reteach: ❑ Return: ❑ Instructor initials: ________

Step 6: Check for a carotid pulse and other signs of circulation.

Yes: ❑ Reteach: ❑ Return: ❑ Instructor initials: ________

Step 7: If no pulse/circulation, begin cycles of 15 compressions to 2 ventilations (rate of 100 compressions per minute). One person may perform both ventilations and compressions until tired and then switch off. Or one rescuer may perform ventilations while the other performs chest compressions.*

Yes: ❑ Reteach: ❑ Return: ❑ Instructor initials: ________

Step 8: After four cycles, reevaluate.

Yes: ❑ Reteach: ❑ Return: ❑ Instructor initials: ________

Step 9: If no change, repeat step 7.

Yes: ❑ Reteach: ❑ Return: ❑ Instructor initials: ________

*If an AED or defibrillator becomes available, stop CPR, analyze the rhythm, and shock as indicated. See Chapter 29 for cardiac arrest emergencies.

Appendix B Skill Sheet

Student Name ______________________________ Date ________________

CPR for a Child—One or Two Rescuers

Step 1: Establish unresponsiveness.

Yes: ❑ Reteach: ❑ Return: ❑ Instructor initials: ________

Step 2: Have the second person obtain an AED or call for advanced assistance.

Yes: ❑ Reteach: ❑ Return: ❑ Instructor initials: ________

Step 3: Open the airway.

Yes: ❑ Reteach: ❑ Return: ❑ Instructor initials: ________

Step 4: Look, listen, and feel.

Yes: ❑ Reteach: ❑ Return: ❑ Instructor initials: ________

Step 5: If no breathing or inadequate breathing, give two slow breaths. (Suction the airway before ventilations, if needed.)

Yes: ❑ Reteach: ❑ Return: ❑ Instructor initials: ________

Step 6: Check for a carotid pulse and other signs of circulation.

Yes: ❑ Reteach: ❑ Return: ❑ Instructor initials: ________

Step 7: If no pulse/circulation, begin cycles of 5 compressions to 1 ventilation (rate of 100 compressions per minute). One person may perform both ventilations and compressions until tired and then switch off. Or one rescuer may perform ventilations while the other performs chest compressions.*

Yes: ❑ Reteach: ❑ Return: ❑ Instructor initials: ________

Step 8: After twenty cycles, reevaluate.

Yes: ❑ Reteach: ❑ Return: ❑ Instructor initials: ________

Step 9: If no change, repeat step 7.

Yes: ❑ Reteach: ❑ Return: ❑ Instructor initials: ________

*If a pediatric AED or defibrillator becomes available, stop CPR, analyze the rhythm, and shock as indicated. See Chapter 39 for pediatric emergencies.

Appendix B Skill Sheet

Student Name ______________________________ Date ________________

CPR for an Infant—One or Two Rescuers

Step 1: Establish unresponsiveness.

Yes: ❑ Reteach: ❑ Return: ❑ Instructor initials: ________

Step 2: Have the second person obtain an AED or call for advanced assistance.

Yes: ❑ Reteach: ❑ Return: ❑ Instructor initials: ________

Step 3: Open the airway.

Yes: ❑ Reteach: ❑ Return: ❑ Instructor initials: ________

Step 4: Look, listen, and feel.

Yes: ❑ Reteach: ❑ Return: ❑ Instructor initials: ________

Step 5: If no breathing or inadequate breathing, give two slow breaths. (Suction the airway before ventilations if needed.)

Yes: ❑ Reteach: ❑ Return: ❑ Instructor initials: ________

Step 6: Check for a brachial pulse and other signs of circulation.

Yes: ❑ Reteach: ❑ Return: ❑ Instructor initials: ________

Step 7: If no pulse/circulation, begin cycles of 5 compressions to 1 ventilation (rate of 100 compressions per minute). One person may perform both ventilations and compressions until tired and then switch off. Or one rescuer may perform ventilations while the other performs chest compressions.*

Yes: ❑ Reteach: ❑ Return: ❑ Instructor initials: ________

Step 8: After 20 cycles, reevaluate.

Yes: ❑ Reteach: ❑ Return: ❑ Instructor initials: ________

Step 9: If no change, repeat step 7.

Yes: ❑ Reteach: ❑ Return: ❑ Instructor initials: ________

*If a pediatric AED or defibrillator becomes available, stop CPR, analyze the rhythm, and shock as indicated. See Chapter 37 for newborn emergencies.

APPENDIX C Advanced Life Support Assist Skills

There are some situations in which the EMT will call for assistance from advanced life support providers. In these circumstances, the EMT may be able to provide support to the ALS unit, if the EMT is familiar with common ALS procedures.

Definitions: Write the definitions of the following terms.

1. laryngoscope ____________________
2. hyperventilation ____________________
3. cricoid pressure ____________________
4. twelve-lead ECG ____________________
5. normal saline (NS) ____________________
6. D5W ____________________
7. macrodrip ____________________
8. lactated Ringers solution (LR) ____________________
9. microdrip ____________________
10. preoxygenation ____________________

Ordering: Place the following steps of preparing IV tubing in the proper sequence by numbering them from 1 to 6.

____ Check the solution for clarity and date.

____ Remove the tab from the solution, and the cap from the drip chamber.

____ Select IV tubing size, open the packaging, and close the roller clamp.

____ Open the roller clamp and allow the fluid through the IV tubing.

____ Put the tubing spike into the appropriate IV solution port on the IV bag.

____ Hold the solution upright, and squeeze the chamber to fill the drip chamber halfway with fluid.

Short Answer: Read each question. Think about the information presented in your text, and then answer each question with one or two sentences.

1. List four key "Do Nots" with regard to handling sharps.

2. Describe at least three ways in which EMTs help an ALS provider intubate a patient successfully.

3. Name and locate correct placement of twelve-lead electrodes on the diagram below.

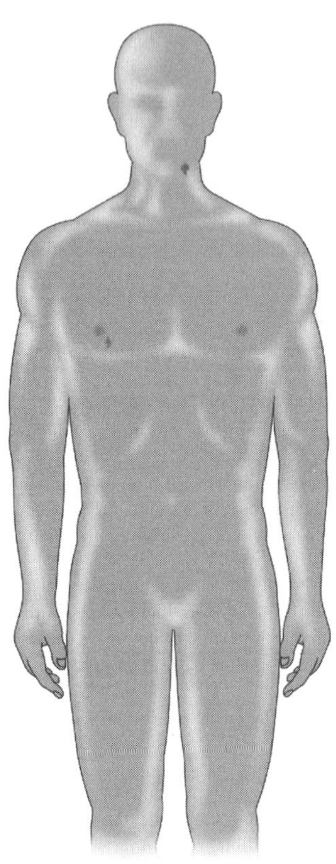

Appendix C Skill Sheet

Student Name ______________________________ Date ______________

Skill C-1: Intravenous Line Preparation

Equipment Needed:

1. Intravenous fluid
2. Intravenous tubing

Yes: ❑ Reteach: ❑ Return: ❑ Instructor initials: ________

Step 1: The EMT verifies that she has the right solution, the solution is not expired, and the solution is clear.

Yes: ❑ Reteach: ❑ Return: ❑ Instructor initials: ________

Step 2: The EMT selects the correct IV tubing, removing it from the box. She moves the roller clamp proximal to the drip chamber and closes the roller clamp.

Yes: ❑ Reteach: ❑ Return: ❑ Instructor initials: ________

Step 3: The EMT removes the tab from the solution, as well as removes the cap from the drip chamber end of tubing.

Yes: ❑ Reteach: ❑ Return: ❑ Instructor initials: ________

Step 4: Without touching either sterile end, the EMT inserts the tubing spike into the appropriate port on the IV bag.

Yes: ❑ Reteach: ❑ Return: ❑ Instructor initials: ________

Step 5: With the bag spiked, the EMT holds the solution upright and squeezes the drip chamber to allow it to fill halfway with solution.

Yes: ❑ Reteach: ❑ Return: ❑ Instructor initials: ________

Step 6: Holding the fluid up with the tubing down, the EMT opens the flow regulator to allow fluid to fill the tubing slowly. The EMT recaps the sterile end once the IV tubing is flushed.

Yes: ❑ Reteach: ❑ Return: ❑ Instructor initials: ________

ANSWER KEY

Chapter 1

Matching:

1. c
2. g
3. j
4. i
5. f
6. e
7. h
8. a
9. d
10. b

True or False:

1. T
2. F
3. F
4. F
5. F
6. F
7. T
8. T
9. F
10. T

Short Answer:

1. Research has shown that trauma patients are best treated within one hour of their injuries. Prehospital care providers quickly remove trauma victims from the scene, assess and treat injuries during transport, and deliver the injured to trauma centers.
2. Military personnel were better trained to provide care to the injured and had better equipment for field stabilization and rapid transport to definitive care at a field hospital. Their civilian counterparts had no standardized training, limited equipment, and most often used hearses or funeral-home-based ambulances for transports.
3. Johnny and Roy raised the expectations that Americans had for prehospital care.
4. Early access, early CPR, early defibrillation, early advanced care.
5. While EMT-Bs play a part in all four components, they play a direct role in early CPR and early defibrillation. EMT-Bs must be advocates for early access by promoting use of 9-1-1 and education regarding recognition and prevention of illnesses and injuries. In many areas of the country, EMT-Bs may actually be the provider requesting advanced level care.
6. Answers will vary.
7. Answers will vary.
8. Answers will vary.

Chapter 2

Ordering:

5 Assess patient
8 Call medical control as needed
7 Continue care during transport
4 Determine mechanism of injury or nature of illness
2 Drive safely to scene
11 Give verbal and written reports to staff
12 Replace any equipment used
6 Move patient to the ambulance
9 Notify destination facility of patient
3 Perform scene assessment
10 Reassess patient
1 Receive information from dispatch

Identification:

X Airway maintenance
X Ventilation of patients
__ Intubation of patients
X CPR
X Defibrillation by AED
__ Manual cardioversion
X Hemorrhage control
__ Suturing of wounds
X Bandaging of wounds
X Assisting in childbirth
__ Prescribing medications to patients

True or False:

1. T
2. F
3. F
4. T
5. F
6. F
7. F

Definitions:

1. certification: proof of satisfactory completion of a course of study
2. medical direction: advice provided by a physician or other higher medical authority
3. off-line medical control: physician involvement in protocol and procedural preparation
4. on-line medical control: direct communication between the EMT-B and physician while care is being given in the field
5. quality management: a continual process involving planning, execution, assessment, review, and improvement of the overall plan
6. professional conduct: behavior demonstrating a caring, confident, and courteous demeanor expected from all health care providers
7. quality improvement: actions taken to improve the quality of care given
8. prehospital health care team: multidisciplinary group composed of medical personnel, firefighters, police officers, and other health professionals who care for patients outside the hospital

Identification:

1. classroom
2. clinical
3. hands-on
4. classroom
5. clinical

Short Answer:

1. By reassuring bystanders, the EMT can reduce the likelihood of misunderstandings, and thus increase the safety for herself and her crew. Additionally, reassurance is a measure provided in an MD's office or hospital. Prehospital care patients and family/friends are entitled to the same level of care. Be careful not to violate the patient's confidentiality.
2. A clean, pressed uniform and clear name tag serve to identify the prehospital care provider. Patients are entitled to know who is caring for them. Also, this will ensure that the provider presents a professional attitude.
3. EMT-Bs must continually practice and update their knowledge and skills, as the field of prehospital emergency care is continually changing due to new research.

Critical Thinking 1:

1. The EMT-Bs have first violated the "Do No Harm" principle, as their conversation may be overheard by others, and can have an effect on their patient's personal life. They have also neglected to hold their patient's information in confidence.
2. Answers will vary.
3. The EMT Code of Ethics lists promoting health as a fundamental responsibility. This may include, but is not limited to, actions such as community health education, health fairs, and working with seniors or other community groups in promoting a healthful lifestyle.

Critical Thinking 2:

1. Planning, execution, assessment, review, and improvements
2. Retrospective quality assessment and prospective quality assessment
3. Retrospective
4. Any answer related to the five elements in answer #1

Critical Thinking 3:

1. Assessment, administration of oxygen, assisting in the self-injection of a medication, transportation, and postcall evaluation
2. Following the directive to change the oxygen administration device
3. While the EMT-Bs are caring for the patient, they are acting as the physician's designated agent.

Chapter 3

Completion:

1. abandonment
2. confidentiality
3. evidence conscious
4. Good Samaritan laws
5. Health care proxy
6. implied consent
7. legal duty to act
8. off-line
9. on-line
10. Bill of Rights
11. pattern of injury
12. restraints
13. causation of injury
14. standard
15. HIPAA

Identification:

1. expressed
2. expressed by parentis loco
3. implied
4. implied by emergency doctrine
5. implied
6. expressed
7. expressed
8. expressed by an emancipated minor

True or False:

1. F
2. F
3. T
4. F
5. F
6. T
7. F
8. F

Identification:

1. duty to act
2. a mistake
3. harm
4. causation of injury
5. a failure to meet standards

Yes or No:

1. NO
2. NO
3. YES
4. NO
5. NO
6. YES
7. NO
8. NO
9. NO
10. YES

Identification:

X Keep unnecessary people off the scene
___ Use the patient's telephone to avoid radio communications
___ Leave all medical materials on the scene
___ Turn off lights
X Remember anything that must be moved for patient care
X Do not touch weapons
X Leave answering machines or caller identification devices alone
___ Cover the body to maintain modesty
X Do not use the sink to wash hands
___ Turn off the TV, radio, and video equipment

Short Answer:

1. The patient must be: an adult, or legally considered to be one; competent; informed of the reasonable and foreseeable consequences of refusal; and he must have been offered care to the limit that he will accept and be encouraged to seek further medical care.
2. By listening carefully, the EMT may hear or sense that the patient is fearful or has not completely understood the information provided.

Critical Thinking 1:

1. Some states permit assessment and/or treatment for pregnancy or sexually transmitted diseases based on the conclusion that providing such early care outweighs the parental right to consent.
2. Parent of a child, in the military, emancipated minor.

Critical Thinking 2:

1. The EMT-Bs need to listen carefully to what Mr. Rotelli is saying and not saying. They should then ask to begin with simple assessment and care, carefully explaining the need for each. They also need to advise Mr. Rotelli that his present condition may be a serious one, resulting in severe illness or death. If they are unable to convince Mr. Rotelli of the advisability of care and transport at this time, they must let him know that they will return at any time, and inform him of any additional medical care provisions in the community.
2. They should contact medical control for advice.
3. They need to document evidence of competence, informed refusal, offers of care to the limit Mr. Rotelli would accept, and the availability of care in the community, including their willingness to return.

Critical Thinking 3:

1. Begin CPR and contact medical control for guidance.

Critical Thinking 4:

1. Observe interactions between the parents and child. Also pay attention to both parents' and child's responses to the EMT-Bs. Note the history given by the parents at different times and any history given by the child.
2. They should report observations only. They should not make judgments or draw conclusions. Report the child's physical condition, including injuries noted, treatment given, and the response to the treatment. Report the behaviors of the child and parents. Report all history given by the child and the parents.

Chapter 4

Missing Letters:

body substance isolation
acute stress
burnout
stress management program
healthy lifestyle
scene survey
stressors
relaxation exercises
multiple casualty incident
fight or flight response
chronic stress
unwind time
stress
diversionary techniques

Matching:

1. b
2. d
3. h
4. e
5. c
6. g
7. a
8. f

Sorting:

Physical	**Emotional**	**Behavioral**
increased heart rate	edgy	avoidance
gastrointestinal distress	depression	withdrawal
anxiety	irritability	aggression
headaches	anger	procrastination
insomnia		alcohol abuse
fatigue		drug abuse
muscle tension		

Short Answer:

1. Prevention of a stressful situation means that the body will not need to physically respond by releasing hormones. Treatment afterward, while important, cannot undo the initial response to the stress hormones.
2. There may be many answers, including cross-training and rotation of assignments.

Critical Thinking 1:

1. Review the situation, including the activity in the ED at the time. Plan how and when to ask questions in the future.
2. Concentrate on goals.
3. Focus on the positives of the care given.

4. Find an aspect of the unit or its staff that is positive and helpful. (Many answers may be acceptable.)

Critical Thinking 2:

1. Yes. Even though this is a positive step, stress occurs from both positive (happy) or negative (sad) events.
2. Liz can try to concentrate on the goal she has achieved. She can focus on the warm wishes of her colleagues. She can begin to plan her practice as a paramedic.

Critical Thinking 3:

1. Long shift, many calls, physical and mental demands, stressed patients and families, pediatric calls, potential exposure to a disease, trauma, an ill child at home
2. Relaxation exercises, physical exercise, engaging in hobbies, travel, social activities

Critical Thinking 4:

1. Stress (physical complaints)
2. The inability of the EMT-B to prevent Mr. Linkowski's death is a significant stressor.
3. Many answers are acceptable. They should include a focus on the positive aspects of Mr. Linkowski's care, care offered to his family, and the steps the EMT-Bs took to make Mr. Linkowski comfortable.

Critical Thinking 5:

1. Joe is experiencing stress related to a previous incident.
2. Joe may experience physical, emotional, and behavioral symptoms/signs.

Chapter 5

Matching:

1. k
2. m
3. g
4. w
5. l
6. h
7. s
8. n
9. r
10. d
11. o
12. x
13. y
14. u
15. f
16. a
17. e
18. j
19. i
20. q
21. p
22. b
23. v
24. t
25. c

Integumentary System
Fill in the Blank:

1. protects
2. epidermis
3. dermis
4. subcutaneous
5. appearance

Muscular System
True or False:

1. T
2. F
3. F
4. F
5. T

Skeletal System
Matching:

1. f
2. a
3. o
4. j
5. i
6. n
7. m
8. k
9. g
10. b
11. c
12. e
13. d
14. h
15. l

Labeling Figure 5-1:

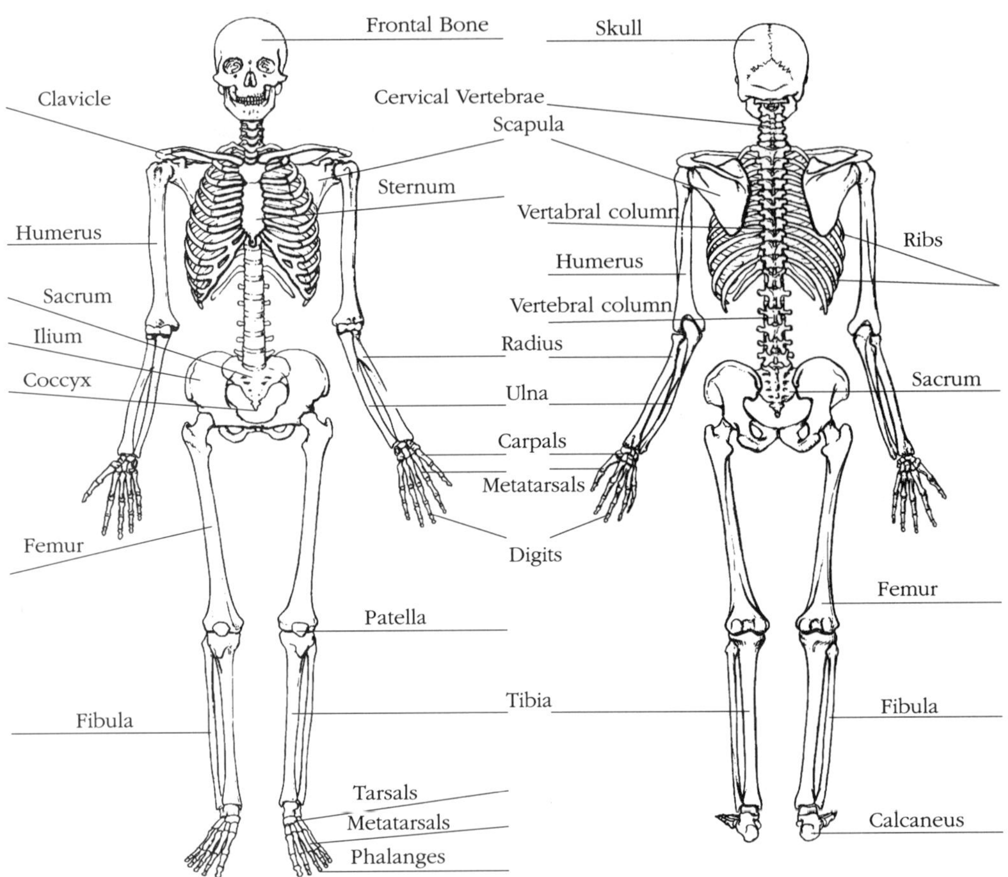

Central Nervous System
Fill in the Blank:
The central nervous system is made up of the BRAIN and the SPINAL CORD. It is involved in the INITIATION and TRANSMISSION of all control messages in the body. The brain consists of the CEREBRUM, the CEREBELLUM, and the BRAINSTEM. The brainstem consists of the MIDBRAIN, PONS, and MEDULLA. The brainstem controls life-sustaining functions such as BREATHING and HEARTBEAT. The "athletic brain" is called the CEREBELLUM. The "athletic brain" controls MUSCULAR COORDINATION. The largest area of the brain, the seat of higher thinking, is called the CEREBRUM. The brain is protected by three membranes called the PIA MATER, ARACHNOID, and the DURA MATER. The brain is also protected by a fluid called CEREBROSPINAL FLUID. The spinal cord begins at the BASE of the SKULL. The PERIPHERAL NERVOUS SYSTEM is made up of nerves that run from the spinal cord to take messages to the body. Automatic functions such as the heart beating are under control of the AUTONOMIC NERVOUS SYSTEM.

Labeling Figure 5-2:

A. ventricle
B. parietal lobe
C. midbrain
D. pons
E. cerebellum
F. medulla oblongata
G. spinal cord
H. skull

Endocrine System
Fill in the Blank:
The ENDOCRINE SYSTEM produces HORMONES, which are chemicals designed to help the nervous system maintain control of the body. The chemicals are produced by organs called GLANDS and are excreted into the BLOODSTREAM. They then affect TARGET organs to change the way the organs function. The pancreas is relevant to the EMT-B because it produces INSULIN that helps the body use GLUCOSE. Diabetics cannot produce this chemical.

Circulatory System

True or False:

1. T
2. F
3. T
4. F
5. F
6. T
7. F
8. T
9. F
10. T

Fill in the Blank:

Beginning at the RIGHT ATRIUM, a drop of blood flows past the TRICUSPID valve and into the right VENTRICLE. From there it passes the PULMONIC valve into the pulmonary ARTERY and onto the lungs. Passing through the pulmonary circulation, the drop of blood returns to the left ATRIUM by the pulmonary VEIN. Moving through the left side of the heart, the blood passes the MITRAL valve into the left VENTRICLE, passes the AORTIC valve and into the AORTA, which is the largest artery in the body. This artery helps deliver blood to body tissues. Oxygen and nutrients are removed, and the blood returns to the right atrium via the VENA CAVA.

Labeling Figure 5-3:

A. apex
B. myocardium
C. Purkinje fibers
D. interventricular spetum
E. superior vena cava
F. inferior vena cava
G. right atrium
H. tricuspid valve
I. right ventricle
J. pulmonary semilunar valve
K. left pulmonary artery
L. left pulmonary veins
M. left atrium
N. bicuspid valve or mitral valve
O. left ventricle
P. aortic semilunar valve
Q. aorta

Respiratory System

Matching:

1. l
2. j
3. n
4. o
5. k
6. h
7. f
8. d
9. b
10. a
11. i
12. e
13. m
14. c
15. g

Labeling Figure 5-4:

A. oral cavity
B. nasal cavity
C. sinuses
D. pharynx
E. esophagus
F. larynx
G. cricoid cartilage
H. trachea
I. left lung
J. right lung
K. bronchi
L. bronchiole
M. alveoli

Digestive System

Fill in the Blank:

The beginning of digestion takes place in the MOUTH. There, the teeth grind the food and allow it to be mixed with SALIVA, a digestive enzyme. The mass of moistened, chewed food is called a BOLUS and it passes the oropharynx and into the ESOPHAGUS, a muscular tube connected to the stomach. There, stomach ACIDS and other enzymes break the food apart. The stomach empties into the SMALL intestine where 90% of the digestion actually takes place. This intestine takes up the largest part of the abdominal cavity. Food then moves into the LARGE intestine, which terminates at the rectum. The rectum forms the feces, or waste products, which are expelled through the anus.

Completion:

Organ	Type	Location	Function
liver	SOLID	RIGHT UPPER QUADRANT	detoxifies poisons
GALLBLADDER	hollow	RIGHT UPPER QUADRANT	stores bile

Organ	Type	Location	Function
pancreas	HOLLOW	center	HORMONES/ENZYMES
appendix	HOLLOW	RIGHT LOWER QUADRANT	unknown
KIDNEYS	solid	retroperitoneal	PRODUCES URINE

Labeling Figure 5-5:

A. oral cavity
B. glands
C. pharynx
D. esophagus
E. liver
F. gallbladder
G. stomach
H. pancreas
I. duodenum
J. small intestine
K. cecum
L. appendix
M. ascending colon
N. large intestine
O. descending colon
P. sigmoid colon
Q. rectum

Reproductive System
Matching:

1. h
2. f
3. d
4. g
5. e
6. c
7. k
8. i
9. b
10. j
11. a

Labeling for Figure 5-6a:

A. scrotum
B. testis
C. epididymis
D. vas deferens
E. seminal vesicle
F. ejaculatory duct
G. prostate gland
H. urethra
I. prepuce
J. glans penis

Labeling for Figure 5-6b:

A. ovary
B. fimbriae of fallopian tube
C. fallopian tube
D. uterus
E. uterine cavity
F. cervix
G. vagina

Chapter 6

Word Scramble:

1. immunization
2. carrier
3. prophylaxis
4. transmission
5. contagious
6. immunocompromise
7. antibody
8. microorganism
9. vector
10. biohazard

Listing:

A. Choose any five examples from Table 6-3 in your text.

B. 1. OSHA 1910.1030
2. NFPA

True or False:

1. F
2. T
3. T
4. F
5. T
6. F
7. T
8. F
9. F
10. T

Definitions:

1. safety officer: a designated person in charge with knowledge of relevant CDC, OSHA, and NFPA regulations regarding safety
2. biohazard: refers to materials considered unsafe because of contamination with body fluids
3. personal protective equipment: gear that may be used by health care providers to protect against exposures or injury
4. immunocompromised: weakened immune state
5. infection control manual: document required of employers outlining risks, procedures, and care for exposures
6. risk profile: likelihood of presence of disease in a certain community

Identification:

X Ongoing health assessment of the EMT.
__ Putting on gloves, gown, and mask before any patient encounter, and then removing what is unnecessary.
X Carrying spare gloves for use with multiple patients.
__ Washing hands only if gloves are unavailable or ripped.
X Using goggles or safety glasses to protect the eyes.
__ Putting on a mask only if you are close to a patient.
X Using a gown for imminent childbirth.
__ Using latex gloves for handling body fluids, and vinyl gloves for patient contact.

Fill in the Blank:

The EMT should first put on FACE and EYE protection. She should then put on the GOWN if it is necessary. Assistance may be needed in TYING the STRINGS in back. Put the GLOVES on last. To remove the PPE, the EMT should go in REVERSE order. Remove the GLOVES. Then reach back and UNTIE or RIP the ties of the GOWN. Turn it inside out and roll it into a ball. Then remove the FACEMASK and EYE protection. Finally, WASH your hands.

Matching:

1. a
2. f
3. b
4. j
5. c
6. g
7. i
8. h
9. d
10. e

Identification:

__ AIDS
__ tuberculosis
X hepatitis B
X rubella
X tetanus
X measles

Identification:

1. airborne
2. vehicle
3. contact
4. vehicle
5. vector
6. contact
7. contact
8. airborne

Short Answer:

1. In order for microorganisms to initiate disease, they must find a portal of entry. Hand washing flushes away microorganisms, preventing their entry into the body or their spread to another person for entry.
2. The EMT may use waterless gel when the hands are not grossly soiled or bloody or when no sink is immediately available.
3. The EMT should perform hand washing with soap and water as soon as sink and running water are available.

Critical Thinking:

1. Remove gloves, wash her hands, and replace the gloves.
2. Use waterless soap or gel if a sink isn't available.
3. Provide any necessary first aid, and follow the *Infection Control Manual* for reporting the incident.
4. If any follow-up care is necessary, it can be started immediately. Also, should it be necessary, Jess's patient is present at the emergency department for further assessment.

Chapter 7

Matching:

1. f
2. h
3. a
4. g
5. j
6. i
7. b
8. e
9. c
10. d

Definitions:

1. ventilation: process of moving air in and out of the lungs
2. apnea: lack of breathing
3. cyanosis: bluish discoloration to the skin
4. epiglottis: cartilaginous structure at the base of the tongue
5. nasal flaring: widening of the nostrils during breathing; indicates respiratory distress, especially in pediatric patients
6. sputum: secretions from the airways
7. sublingual: under the tongue
8. gag reflex: protective response when the back of the throat is stimulated
9. occlusion: a blockage
10. Yankauer tip: rigid suction catheter with a curve and large open tip

Identification:

X apnea
X cyanosis
X breathlessness
__ cough
X snoring
__ intact dentures
__ conjunctiva
__ uvula
__ sneezing

Ordering:

5 Maintain open airway during entire call
4 Avoid pressure on underside of the jaw
1 Kneel at the level of the head
3 Push down on the forehead and lift up on the chin
2 Place the palm of one hand on the forehead and the fingertips on the jaw

Identification:

1. NPA
2. OPA
3. NPA
4. OPA
5. OPA
6. OPA
7. NPA

Correcting:

1. Suctioning removes debris and air.
2. Open, assess, suction, and secure the airway.
3. Suction to the depth of the measurement taken.
4. Adequate suctioning will take 15 seconds per attempt.
5. Apply suction while withdrawing the catheter.
6. Use a Yankauer catheter to suction blood.
7. French catheters are best for suctioning a tracheostomy.
8. Measure the depth of suctioning from the opening of the mouth to the angle of the jaw.
9. Flush catheters between each suction attempt.
10. It is necessary to wear gloves when suctioning. (Facemask and eyewear too!)

Critical Thinking:

1. They must have PPE, barrier devices, oxygen, suction, and airway-assistive devices.
2. Tania and Geoff should put on facemask, eye protection, and gloves.
3. Unconsciousness and snoring
4. Jaw thrust; no one saw what happened, and trauma cannot be ruled out.

5. Once the airway is opened, assess, suction, and secure.
6. An OPA must be done.
7. Geoff must continue to monitor the airway, as the body needs a continuous source of oxygen.

Chapter 8

Matching:

1. g	6. l	11. d
2. m	7. b	12. e
3. k	8. a	13. j
4. n	9. o	14. i
5. f	10. c	15. h

Identification:

1. Accessory muscles
2. Auscultate
3. Cricoid pressure
4. Intercostal muscles
5. Humidification
6. Dead space
7. Nasal cannula
8. Non-rebreather mask
9. Pursed lip breathing
10. Tracheostomy or stoma

Identification:

X seesaw breathing	__ cricoid pressure	X tripod
X air hunger	__ apex	__ uvula
X pursed lip breathing	X accessory muscle use	__ sneezing

Short Answer:

1. 21% oxygen
2. Moving a gas (air) in and out of the lungs
3. Adding or ensuring that oxygen is the gas moving in and out of the lungs
4. Yes. Another gas; for example, carbon monoxide could move in and out of the lungs. Because it displaces oxygen, it would not help the patient.

Identification:

1. Pocket mask
2. Bag-valve-mask (BVM)
3. Flow-restricted oxygen-powered ventilation device (FROPVD)
4. Non-rebreather mask (NRB)
5. Trach mask
6. Humidification tubing
7. Nasal cannula (NC)

Short Answer:

1. There is increased flammability in the presence of oxygen.
2. Petroleum products may ignite.
3. Extreme temperatures cause pressure changes in the tank. This could cause an explosion.
4. Modified regulators may lead to leaks and they will fail to identify the gas in the cylinder.
5. The tank may empty, leaving the patient at risk for hypoxia.
6. A tank may fall over. At least, it can injure a patient or EMT. If the neck of the tank breaks, it could explode.

Critical Thinking:

1. Posture, effort, accessory muscle use, mental status
2. Number of words spoken per breath, effort, patient's own description of problem
3. Tripod position, conservation of words, pursed lip breathing
4. They should assess the airway for patency, listen to the lungs, palpate the chest wall, observe any accessory muscle use, and assess the skin for color and condition. Additionally, they need an estimate of the breathing rate.
5. Ausculate
6. Mr. Allen is having respiratory distress.
7. Approximately 80–90%

8. Monitor for any changes, including a decrease in his level of response and the development of any secretions that may block the airway.
9. There is no need to place an assistive device at this time, but since Mr. Allen is awake, the EMTs could place an NPA first if the need for one arises. They could change to an OPA if he loses consciousness.

Chapter 9

Missing Letters:

hemorrhagic shock
hypovolemia
PASG
stroke volume
decompensated
evisceration
irreversible shock
perfusion
urticaria
septic shock
cardiogenic shock
cardiac output
neurogenic shock

Identification:

1. Hemorrhagic
2. Hypovolemic
3. Hypovolemic
4. Hypovolemic
5. Anaphylactic
6. Septic
7. Anaphylactic
8. Neurogenic
9. Cardiogenic

Ordering:

3 brain
2 abdominal organs
1 skin, muscles, bones, and uterus
4 heart and lungs

Identification:

1. compensated
2. decompensated
3. decompensated
4. compensated
5. compensated
6. compensated
7. compensated
8. decompensated

True or False:

1. F
2. T
3. F
4. F
5. T
6. F
7. T
8. F
9. T
10. F

Short Answer:

1. Anaphylactic, septic, neurogenic
2. Hypovolemia, hemorrhagic (a type of hypovolemic)
3. Cardiogenic
4. No, removal of PASG/MAST is based on volume replacement that the EMT cannot do.
5. Every 5 minutes

Critical Thinking 1:

1. Does Brittany appear sick? What is her mental status? How is her respiratory status? What is her skin color? How long is capillary refill time?
2. This gives a good indication of Brittany's mental status.
3. Children can compensate very well for decreased perfusion. By the time the BP drops in pediatric patients, shock is well advanced.
4. Supplemental oxygen, position the child flat, legs may be elevated as long as there are no contraindications, prevent heat loss, transport, call for ALS.

Critical Thinking 2:

1. Tilt test, to check for orthostatic vital signs
2. Supplemental oxygen, position the patient in Trendelenburg as long as there are no contraindications, prevent heat loss, transport, call for ALS

Critical Thinking 3:

1. Hypotension (low BP)
2. Urticaria (hives)
3. Supplemental oxygen, position the patient in Trendelenburg as long as there are no contraindications, prevent heat loss, transport, call for ALS, and search for epinephrine prescribed for the patient. Do not delay transport to search extensively.

Chapter 10

Definitions:

1. anisocoria: unequal pupils
2. cyanosis: bluish skin
3. constricted: small/tight
4. jaundice: yellowish skin color
5. dilated: widened
6. pallor: pale skin color
7. diastolic: bottom number of the BP; reflects pressure in the vessels when the heart is at rest
8. PERRL: pupils equal, round, reactive to light
9. systolic: top number of the BP, reflects pressure when the heart contracts
10. sphygmomanometer: device to measure BP

Matching:

1. e
2. h
3. g
4. b
5. i
6. c
7. f
8. j
9. d
10. a

Calculation of respiratory rates:

1. 30 breaths per minute
2. 20 breaths per minute
3. 24 breaths per minute
4. 12 breaths per minute

Calculation of pulse rates:

1. 64 beats per minute
2. 90 beats per minute
3. 68 beats per minute
4. 90 beats per minute
5. 104 beats per minute

True or False:

1. F
2. T
3. F
4. T
5. F

Sorting:

Color	**Temperature**	**Condition**
pink	cool	sweaty
pallor	hot	dry
cyanosis	warm	
jaundice		
flushed		
gray		

Identification:

1. sign
2. symptom
3. symptom
4. sign
5. sign
6. sign
7. symptom
8. sign
9. sign
10. sign
11. symptom
12. symptom
13. sign
14. sign
15. symptom

Sorting:

S "difficulty breathing"
tripod
accessory muscle use
A eggs
M Ventolin
vitamins
aspirin
P lung disease
L breakfast this AM
last used inhaler 1 hour ago
E smoker
hot/humid

Chapter 11

Definitions:

1. firefighter's drag
2. rescuer assist
3. arm drag
4. pack strap carry
5. diamond stretcher carry
6. seat carry
7. end-to-end stretcher carry
8. caterpillar pass
9. squat lift
10. firefighter's carry
11. power lift
12. clothing drag
13. direct lift
14. emergency moves
15. direct carry
16. blanket drag
17. cradle carry
18. extremity carry

Matching:

1. c
2. g
3. b
4. h
5. f
6. a
7. d
8. e

Identification:

1. __ Person stuck in a car; complaining of leg pain
2. X Person unconscious from smoke in a fireworks factory
3. X Person with a fractured leg is lying across a patient in respiratory arrest
4. __ The driver of a car smashed her face and knocked out several teeth; airway patent
5. X Person is still inside a vehicle which has overturned into a creek
6. __ A person is complaining of back and leg pain
7. __ A person has bleeding from a head laceration
8. __ A person is complaining of mild shortness of breath following a fender bender
9. X A person collapses outside a building where there is a gas leak
10. X A person is in respiratory arrest following a minor accident

Short Answer:

1. Lumbar spine
2. Strengthening exercises for back and abdominal muscles
3. Squat down close to the tools. Pull them toward your body. Holding the tools close to your body, stand straight up using the large muscles of your legs. Do not bend or twist.
4. Use a draw sheet to pull the patient toward you onto the stretcher, or use a slide or transfer board.
5. Wearing the device tightly and at all times can lead to a weakening of the back muscles.

Critical Thinking:

1. Scoop stretcher or flexible stretcher can be used in the tight quarters.
2. An emergency move not requiring the use of the patient's arms. A clothing drag or blanket drag would work in this circumstance.
3. Any method that can keep Mrs. Hedderman sitting upright. The stair chair is safe and easy, but in a pinch, a chair carry would work. Ted and Katie must be assured of Mrs. Hedderman's safety if they use the chair carry.

Chapter 12

Completion:

1. The INITIAL REPORT is the first radio report of the scene conditions.
2. The feeling that there is an increased likelihood of injury is based on a HIGH INDEX of SUSPICION.
3. A device intended to produce death is a(n) DEADLY WEAPON, while one capable of death or serious harm in certain circumstances is a(n) DANGEROUS INSTRUMENT.
4. The PERIMETER divides hazardous areas from nonhazardous areas. A barrier that protects EMTs and permits them to work is a(n) SAFETY CORRIDOR.
5. A scene SURVEY must be done to determine if any hazards are on-scene. Emergency vehicles can then be STAGED safely in a specific place.

Identification:

1. loaded, extent of damage
2. crumple zone
3. doors locked or jammed, windows open or broken, intrusion into body
4. cracks, starred
5. air bag deployment, mirror broken, seat belts used, wheel bent, headrest broken, cracked dash, pedals bent, seat knocked off pedestal, intrusion
6. fluids leaking

Identification:

__	Enter a car sitting on its roof	__	Close windows
X	Take the transmission out of drive	__	Cut seat belts
X	Turn off the engine	X	Engage parking brake
__	Chock the wheels		

True or False:

1.	F	6.	T
2.	T	7.	F
3.	F	8.	T
4.	F	9.	T
5.	T	10.	T

Correcting:

1. Replace "operations" with "incident command management"
2. Replace "scene survey" with "staging"
3. Replace "cannot" with "can"
4. Remove the words "two times"

Short Answer:

1.	Broken rearview mirror	forehead
2.	Bent steering wheel	torso
3.	Broken dash	knees
4.	Seat knocked off pedestal	body
5.	Locked seat belt	torso

Critical Thinking 1:
The dry powder, spilled gas, angry patrons, curious onlookers, traffic

Critical Thinking 2:
High speed traffic, curiosity, loaded bumpers, antifreeze or fuel leaking onto ground, flares igniting fuels

Critical Thinking 3:
Poor lighting, lack of repairs, animals, guns

Chapter 13

Identification:

__	an injured, deformed leg	X	a stab wound to the chest
X	vomit in the mouth	X	absent radial pulse
__	history of a heart attack	__	allergy to penicillin
X	crepitus over the neck and chest	X	snoring respirations
__	a bone deformed in the arm	X	blood-soaked jeans
__	gives a complete medical history	__	breakfast last eaten
__	use of cocaine	X	tenderness of chest wall

Identification:

1. A
2. U
3. V
4. P
5. A
6. A
7. V
8. V
9. P

Sorting:

Patent	Nonpatent
quiet breathing	snoring
speaking clearly	unresponsive
alert and oriented	vomitus
good chest rise	broken teeth in mouth
	infant unable to cry
	drooling
	stridor
	very bloody nose

True or False:

1. F
2. T
3. T
4. T
5. T
6. T
7. F
8. F
9. T
10. F
11. T

Definitions:

1. alert: awake and interacting with the environment
2. crepitus: the feeling of air under the skin; feels like Rice Krispies
3. sternal rub: rubbing the knuckles against the patient's sternum
4. flail chest: two or more ribs broken in two or more places, resulting in a free floating section of the ribcage
5. paradoxical motion: movement of the flail segment opposite to the rest of the chest wall
6. AVPU: acronym to remember the classes of mental status
7. ABCs: the technique of assessing airway, breathing, and circulation in order
8. unresponsive: cannot be aroused with verbal or painful stimuli

Short Answer:

1. The EMT can determine whether there is trauma or a medical complaint; whether the patient appears sick or not sick, and how fast the team should be moving.
2. The EMT must obtain information about rate and adequacy.
3. The EMT must control bleeding that is excessive in amount or potentially life threatening.

Identification:

1. high
2. low
3. low
4. high
5. low
6. high
7. high
8. high
9. low

Critical Thinking 1:

1. The patient is unresponsive.
2. Since the patient is unresponsive, the EMT should presume that the airway is not patent.
3. Assign this patient high priority.

Critical Thinking 2:

1. No, there is not a potentially life-threatening condition present.
2. They know his airway is patent, and his breathing adequate for speech.
3. Assign this patient low priority.

Critical Thinking 3:

1. Yes; a complicated childbirth, and shock, are potentially life threatening.
2. They should anticipate that it will be inadequate.
3. Assign this patient high priority.

Chapter 14

Word Scramble:

1. abrasion
2. burn
3. contusion
4. deformity
5. guarding
6. laceration
7. puncture
8. swelling
9. tender
10. crepitus

True or False:

1. F
2. T
3. T
4. T
5. T
6. T
7. F
8. F
9. F
10. T

Listing:

1. Be polite
2. Give explanations
3. Maintain privacy
4. Make eye contact
5. Be honest
6. Focus the patient's attention

Identification:

X Vehicle rollover with unrestrained patient
__ Fall of 10 feet
X Death of another occupant in the vehicle
__ Farm trauma
__ Vehicle-pedestrian accident
X Twenty inches of front-end damage
X Ejection
__ Motorcycle accident
X Crash speed of 20 mph or greater

Ordering:

5 Obtain baseline vitals signs
7 Document
1 Size-up/scene safety
6 Obtain a SAMPLE history
2 Complete an initial assessment, including spinal precautions
3 Consider ALS
4 Complete a rapid trauma assessment

Completion:

See Table 14-3 in text book.
The acronym reminds the EMT-B to search for serious underlying injury.

Critical Thinking 1:

1. minor
2. size-up/scene safety; initial, focused trauma assessment; vital signs; SAMPLE

Critical Thinking 2:

1. major
2. size-up/scene safety; initial, rapid trauma assessment; vital signs; SAMPLE

Critical Thinking 3:

1. major
2. size-up/scene safety; initial, rapid trauma assessment; vital signs; SAMPLE

Critical Thinking 4:

1. minor
2. size-up/scene safety; initial, focused trauma assessment; vital signs; SAMPLE

Critical Thinking 5:

1. minor
2. size-up/scene safety; initial, focused trauma assessment; vital signs; SAMPLE

Chapter 15

Matching:

1. a
2. f
3. e
4. b
5. h
6. c
7. d
8. g

True or False:

1. T
2. F
3. T
4. T
5. F
6. F
7. T
8. F
9. F
10. T

Ordering:

4 Rapid trauma exam
2 First impression
1 Scene survey/size-up
5 Detailed exam
3 Initial exam

Listing:

skull: DCAP-BTLS, plus extent of bleeding, remove glass shards
ears: DCAP-BTLS, presence of drainage, Battle's sign

eyes:	DCAP-BTLS, raccoon eyes, size, shape and reaction to light, foreign material, accumulation of blood in the anterior chamber
face:	DCAP-BTLS
nose:	DCAP-BTLS, bleeding, CSF drainage, mucous drainage
mouth:	DCAP-BTLS, dentures or dental appliances, hoarseness to the voice, stability of teeth, bleeding
neck:	DCAP-BTLS, position of the trachea
chest:	DCAP-BTLS, crepitus, paradoxical motion, shallow breathing, lung sounds
abdomen:	DCAP-BTLS, distension, seat belt signs, urinary incontinence
extremities:	DCAP-BTLS, symmetry, pulses, movement, sensation

Critical Thinking 1:

1. Life threats
2. CSF drainage from the ears or nose; changes in pupil size, shape or responses; DCAP-BTLS of the head, neck, and back

Critical Thinking 2:

1. Abdominal distension, tenderness beneath the reddened areas
2. An abdominal injury with possible hypoperfusion

Chapter 16

Sorting:

S	headache shortness of breath	**P**	asthma eczema
A	hives with penicillin wheezing after eating nuts	**L**	asthma attack 1 week ago ate breakfast
M	Ventolin q6 hours aspirin daily Theo-Dur QID	**E**	cleaning with bleach

Ordering:

8	Ongoing assessment	3	OPQRST
2	Chief complaint	1	Initial assessment
4	SAMPLE	7	Treat and transport
6	Baseline vital signs	5	Focused physical exam

Ordering:

4	SAMPLE history	3	Baseline vital signs
1	Initial assessment	2	Rapid physical exam
5	Treat and transport	6	Ongoing assessment

Short Answer:

1. unresponsive medical
2. trauma insignificant mechanism
3. trauma significant mechanism
4. responsive medical
5. trauma insignificant mechanism
6. trauma significant mechanism
7. responsive medical
8. unresponsive medical
9. trauma significant mechanism
10. responsive medical

Definitions:

1. chief complaint: the patient's main problem and the reason for calling
2. focused physical exam: physical exam focused upon the chief complaint
3. medic alert bracelet: a bracelet worn by those with chronic medical problems
4. ongoing assessment: the continued observation of the patient throughout contact
5. on-line medical control: speaking directly with the MD while caring for the patient

6. OPQRST: a device used to prompt questions related to the chief complaint
7. SAMPLE: a device to prompt questions regarding the patient's history
8. vial of life: plastic container with a listing of essential medical information

True or False:

1. T
2. F
3. T
4. T
5. T
6. F
7. F
8. T
9. F

Critical Thinking 1:

1. Medical alert jewelry, vial of life, family or bystanders
2. This patient would be considered a high priority, and transport should be initiated at the end of the initial assessment.

Critical Thinking 2:

1. The headache is the chief complaint; it is the reason for the EMS call.

Chapter 17

Short Answer:

1. Identify significant changes in the patient's condition, and evaluate effectiveness of care.
2. The ongoing assessment is begun after the patient has been thoroughly assessed, vital signs have been measured, and a transport decision has been made; also, the history and physical exams have been completed.

Identification:

X mental status
X airway
__ SAMPLE
__ baseline vital signs
X breathing
X empty oxygen tank
X pulse oximetry
X distal pulses
__ history
X pulses
X effectiveness of meds
__ home safety
__ abrasions to forearms
X bleeding
X pulse, respirations, BP

Critical Thinking:

1. Pulse has increased, mental status has changed, patient condition has deteriorated, priority is high
2. Respiratory rate has dropped, effort has decreased, patient condition has improved, priority remains high
3. Mental status has deteriorated, priority is high

Chapter 18

Definitions:

1. base station: original radio transmitters
2. communications center: dispatch
3. communications specialist: the dispatcher
4. med channel: 10 frequencies used nationwide for communications between ambulances and physicians
5. tactical channel: frequency used for nondispatch communications
6. trunked line: system using computers to triage frequencies

Matching:

1. g
2. o
3. h
4. n
5. m
6. a
7. l
8. k
9. b
10. c
11. f
12. i
13. e
14. j
15. d

Listing:

1. telephone interrogation
2. triage
3. dispatch
4. logistics
5. resource networking
6. prearrival instructions

Identification:

1. two-way radio
2. base station
3. mobile radio
4. repeater
5. portable radio
6. simplex
7. duplex

Sorting:

B unit identifier
B ETA
B mental status
B treatments in progress
C exam findings
B age/gender
B chief complaint
B vital signs
C SAMPLE
C changes after treatments

Short Answer:

1. They are able to prioritize 9-1-1 calls in order to only send units with red lights and siren when absolutely necessary. They are also able to give callers instructions over the telephone, with regard to medical emergencies.
2. Prioritizing of 9-1-1 calls, telephone assistance, and prearrival instructions.
3. They are able to give medical assistance via the telephone.
4. The FCC regulates all communications and radio usage throughout the country.

Critical Thinking:

Alert Report:
Medical Center, this is Action Rescue Squad 1.
En route to your facility with a 70-year-old female who is complaining of a headache.
Vital signs are: respirations 16 and nonlabored, pulse 64 and regular, BP 198/98
We have the patient on high-flow oxygen and have requested an ALS intercept.
ETA is 20 minutes.

Consultation Report:
Medical Center, this is BLS Action Rescue Squad 1.
En route to your facility with a 70-year-old female who is complaining of a headache.
Neighbors indicate that the patient is not acting right today, although was all right last evening.
Patient is unable to answer to simple questions. She has no known allergies, is taking medication for a history of high blood pressure and glaucoma, and also takes an aspirin daily.
We cannot determine compliance with medications or time of last meal.
Patient is alert on AVPU scale.
Vital signs are: respirations 16 and nonlabored, pulse 64 and regular, BP 198/98
There is a droop to her mouth when she smiles, and left-hand grasp is much weaker than the right.
We have the patient on high-flow oxygen and have requested an ALS intercept.
There has been no change in patient complaint or condition since applying the oxygen.
Our ETA is 20 minutes.

Chapter 19

Definitions:

1. abandonment: leaving a patient's side prior to the completion of care
2. confidentiality: keeping conversations regarding patient information at a professional status
3. repetitive persistence: rephrase the same statement over and over again, until the patient understands
4. verbal report: a report given to the bedside nurse, or a doctor or nurse over the radio

Listing:

1. Person
2. Place
3. Time

Critical Thinking 1:

1. She is not a nurse, she doesn't work at the hospital, and she is not the nurse for that patient.
2. Introduce himself to the person; ask whom to give report to.

Critical Thinking 2:

1. Make eye contact; ask the nurse directly if she needs any further information regarding the patient.

Critical Thinking 3:

1. The patient can describe his condition more clearly; the nurse would prefer first-hand information.
2. All information included in the medical report should be given to the nurse at the time of patient turnover.

Chapter 20

True or False:

1. T
2. T
3. T
4. F
5. F
6. F
7. T
8. F

Fill in the Blank:

1. affidavit
2. objective
3. plan
4. subjective observation
5. objective
6. subjective
7. objective
8. special incident report

Listing:

1. Quality improvement
2. Legal document
3. Ambulance corps and/or state records
4. Research

Short Answer:

1. The closed format PCR has check-off boxes or bubbles for the EMT to fill. Patient information must conform to the boxes or bubbles. The open format allows the EMT to document observations in longhand.
2. It is useful for large quantities of data.
3. It allows for individual documentation.

Critical Thinking:

SOAP

S C/C hurts to breathe
Patient states the motor vehicle collision occurred due to cell phone distraction
Allergy to penicillin
Takes a pill for high blood pressure
Has history of high blood pressure
Had hernia surgery 3 years ago
Just finished lunch
Denies loss of consciousness

O 40 mph posted speed
No skid marks observed
Restrained driver and only occupant
Steering wheel intact
Air bag deployed
A on AVPU
Speaking in 2–3 words per breath
Respirations 26 per minute and shallow
Tenderness over chest wall
Lung sounds clear
Vital signs BP 116/76 and pulse 100 and regular
Motor, sensory, and circulation intact

A Shortness of breath
Chest trauma
Potential C-spine injury

P C-spine stabilization
C-collar
High-flow oxygen
Short spine board to long spine board
Transport to trauma center
Reassess after movement and q5 minutes during transport

CHEATED
C "Hurts to breathe"
H Restrained driver, single occupant, struck tree
40 mph posted speed
No skid marks noted
No steering wheel deformity
Positive air bag deployment
S Grimace
Shallow breathing
2–3 words per breath
A Penicillin
M BP pill
P High blood pressure
Hernia surgery 3 years ago
L Lunch just prior to event
E Motor vehicle collision due to cell phone use per patient
E A on AVPU
Airway clear
Lung sounds clear
Positive distal pulses
No apparent bleeding
Chest wall tenderness without deformity
Speaking 2–3 words per breath
No deformities of arms or legs
Motor, sensory, and circulation intact
A Shortness of breath
Chest trauma
Potential C-spine injury
T C-spine stabilization
C-collar
High-flow oxygen
Short spine board to long spine board
E Motor, sensory, and circulation after move
Ongoing assessment q5 minutes
D Transport to trauma center
(turn over comments here)

Chapter 21

Matching:

1. g
2. h
3. j
4. a
5. f
6. b
7. d
8. i
9. e
10. c

Identification:

1. Battle's sign
2. Otorrhea
3. Raccoon eyes
4. Rhinorrhea
5. Cushing's triad

True or False:

1. F
2. T
3. F
4. T
5. T
6. F
7. T
8. T
9. T
10. F

Calculation:

1. 3/2/4 = 9
2. 4/5/6 = 15
3. 1/1/2 = 4
4. 1/1/1 = 3
5. 3/4/5 = 12

Sorting:

X ventilate at up to 20 breaths per minute in the adult patient
X elevate the head of the stretcher or board
__ stop CSF flow
X control bleeding
__ determine exact diagnosis
__ withhold oxygen
X provide rapid transport
__ avoid helicopter transport due to pressure changes
X calculate GCS

Fill in the Blank:
The most important thing an EMT can do to improve the outcome of a head-injured patient is to adequately assess and manage the AIRWAY, BREATHING, and CIRCULATORY status. The brain needs adequate perfusion with well-OXYGENATED blood. After ensuring an adequate airway, assess the effectiveness of the patient's own BREATHING. Next, turn attention to the CIRCULATORY status.

For the patient who has suffered a significant injury, the EMT should then move on to a RAPID TRAUMA ASSESSMENT. For a high-priority patient, this will be done during transport. During both assessments completed up to this time, the LEVEL of CONSCIOUSNESS, or patient responsiveness, will be observed. This can be quantified on the GLASGOW COMA scale. A TREND or pattern that may be seen in repeated vital signs is an increased BP, decreased pulse rate, and changed respiratory pattern. This combination is called CUSHING'S TRIAD.

As with all high priority patients, be sure the patient is receiving high-FLOW OXYGEN. Ongoing assessments should be completed every 5 minutes.

Short Answer:
1. Swelling in the head makes it difficult for blood to flow to brain cells. An adequate or somewhat higher blood pressure is needed to overcome the swelling that has occurred. Hypotension in the head injured patient means that little to no blood will reach the brain cells.
2. The fontaneles are areas where the bones have not yet grown together and fused. Any swelling of brain tissue will seek an "escape" route and push through the open areas of the bones.

Critical Thinking 1:
1. Head, spine, and limb injuries are most likely.
2. They must provide C-spine stabilization, control the airway, provide oxygen and ventilate as necessary, and control any external bleeding.
3. AVPU and Glasgow Coma Scale
4. They can elevate the head of the spine board slightly to facilitate venous drainage, and they can oxygenate/ventilate.

Critical Thinking 2:
1. They must provide C-spine stabilization, control the airway, provide oxygen, and ventilate as necessary. If there was any external bleeding, they would need to control that as well.
2. Decreasing mental status, persistent vomiting, a Glasgow Coma Scale score of less than 8, unequal pupils, seizures, hypertension, bradycardia, changes in respiratory pattern
3. Surgical intervention

Chapter 22

Word Scramble:
1. paralysis
2. paraplegia
3. paresthesia
4. quadriplegia
5. priapism

Identification:
1. vertebrae
2. cervical
3. thoracic
4. lumbar
5. meninges

Fill in the Blank:
The first clue the EMT has as to the possibility of a spinal injury is the MECHANISM of INJURY. Knowing the stacked nature of the vertebrae will enable the EMT to imagine the injuries. In a motor vehicle collision, the most common injury type is FLEXION/EXTENSION of the neck. Falls can result in BROKEN bones that intrude into the cord, or COMPRESSION fractures that actually crush the vertebrae. The phenomenon, known as AXIAL LOADING, can cause trauma along the spinal column, especially in the lumbar region. Firearms can lead to spinal injuries due to the uncertainty of the DIRECTION of TRAVEL of the bullet. Sports injuries may also cause spinal injury.

True or False:

1. F
2. T
3. T
4. T
5. F
6. F
7. T
8. F
9. F
10. F

Short Answer:

1. The patient can suffer bone or ligament injuries that do not impinge on the cord. The patient should not be allowed to continue walking around, as these injuries make the column unstable and the cord susceptible to damage.
2. The patient has injured his coccyx. He has not sustained cord damage, however, as the cord ends at the second lumbar region.
3. The injury in the cervical region can impair messages from the respiratory center to the diaphragm.
4. There are no messages to the heart or blood vessels. This results in the heart not speeding up or the vessels redirectly flow away from the skin.
5. The EMT should try to avoid a head-tilt/chin-lift. Use a jaw thrust instead.

Critical Thinking:

1. Manual stabilization of spine; C-collar; short spinal device; to long spine board
2. Manual stabilization of spine; C-collar; rapid extrication to a long spine board
3. Manual stabilization of spine; C-collar; standing takedown to a long spine board

Chapter 23

Missing Letters:

cardiac contusion
hemoptysis
evisceration
sucking chest wound
tamponade
hemothorax
abdomen
paradoxical motion
pulmonary contusion
subcutaneous emphysema
flail segment
tension pneumothorax
petechiae
tracheal deviation

Identification:

B Subcutaneous emphysema
B Tachycardia
B Tachypnea
B Difficulty breathing
B Diminished breath sounds
T Jugular venous distension
T Loss of radial pulses
T Decreased lung compliance
T Hypotension
T Tracheal deviation

Labeling: See Figure 23-1 in your text.

Completion:

1. blunt
2. bleeding
3. pain, breathing
4. DCAP-BTLS
5. subcutaneous emphysema
6. oxygenation, perfusion
7. hemothorax
8. occlusive dressing
9. three
10. affected

True or False:

1. T
2. T
3. F
4. F
5. F
6. F
7. F
8. T
9. T
10. T

Short Answer:

1. The treatment is the same. Trying to accurately diagnose takes time that could be better spent on speedy packaging. Recognition of abdominal trauma is the most important responsibility.
2. Covering with a moist sterile dressing offers protection from infection, saves the area from drying out, and conserves heat.

Critical Thinking:

1. They know he is alert, has an open airway at present, is breathing sufficiently well to enable him to yell, and his brain is sufficiently perfused to allow him to sit up and think through things.
2. While he was shot in the chest, it is a dynamic space. There is the potential for lung, rib, liver, and small intestine damage. Bone fragments from any shattered bone could also cause wider damage.
3. They should provide high-flow oxygen and closely monitor respirations. If necessary, be ready to ventilate. Cover the wound with an occlusive dressing. Call for ALS intercept if available.
4. Transport the patient on his affected side.
5. Open one side of the occlusive dressing. It is possible that covering the wound site allowed air to become trapped and pressure to be built up, creating a tension pneumothorax.

Chapter 24

Missing Letters:

stellate

OSHA

rein**f**orce

tattooing

trauma dressing

rule of n**i**nes

stridor

spiral bandage

wo**u**nd

tourniqu**e**t

un**i**versal dressing

tria**n**gular dressing

straddle in**j**ury

punct**u**re

supe**r**ficial burn

occlus**i**ve dressing

Palm**e**r method

pres**s**ure dressing

Identification:

1. cravat
2. bandage
3. gauze
4. triangle
5. dressing
6. trauma
7. pressure dressing
8. figure 8
9. occlusive
10. compress
11. recurrent dressing
12. roller bandage
13. spiral bandage
14. universal dressing
15. tourniquet

Definitions:

1. hemorrhage: a medical term for excessive bleeding
2. inflammation: the body's attempt to prevent infection and begin healing
3. necrotic: dead tissue
4. coagulation: the process of blood clotting
5. ecchymosis: a wider collection of blood under the skin caused by a rupture of a large blood vessel
6. fasciotomy: a surgical procedure whereby the skin is cut to relieve pressure

True or False:

1. T
2. F
3. F
4. F
5. F
6. T
7. T
8. F

Sorting:

Arterial bleeding	Venous bleeding	Capillary bleeding
spurting	constant	watery
pulsing	deep red	seeping
bright red	pouring out of wound	oozing
	rivulets	

Calculation:

1. 18%
2. 27%
3. 28%
4. 1–1.5%
5. 18%
6. 1%
7. 18%
8. 31.5%
9. 1%
10. 4.5%

Identification:

1. superficial
2. superficial
3. full thickness
4. partial thickness
5. full thickness
6. full thickness
7. full thickness
8. full thickness
9. partial thickness
10. superficial

Short Answer:

1. Blistering opens the skin, permitting germs to enter. Also, the patient was around equipment that may have been unclean.
2. There is no way to determine the exact trajectory of the bullet. Additionally, other injuries that may have occurred in conjunction with the GSW may lead to patient decompensation.
3. The object may be preventing a loss of blood. Removing it would allow the blood to flow freely.
4. Bleeding from the cheek can be controlled from both outside and inside the mouth. It is difficult to control the airway with an object impaled into the cheek.

Critical Thinking 1:

1. Airway and bleeding
2. Airway management, high-flow oxygen, occlusive dressing to the wound, bleeding control
3. Mark remains at risk for an air embolism, which would interfere with blood flow and could lead to hypoxia.

Critical Thinking 2:

1. A sucking chest wound
2. Respiratory distress
3. Airway management, high-flow oxygen, ventilate as needed, occlusive dressing to the chest wound, bleeding control

Chapter 25

Identification:

1. Humerus, radius, ulna
2. Carpals, metacarpals, and phalanges
3. Femur, patella, tibia, and fibula
4. Tarsals, matatarsals, calcaneus, phalanges
5. Scapula, clavicles, ribs, sternum, vertebrae, pelvis

Definitions:

1. closed fracture: a broken bone in which the bone ends do not break the skin
2. dislocation: a bone that slips out of the joint, out of alignment
3. dorsiflexion: movement of the toes upward toward the nose
4. footdrop: a loss of nervous control that results in a flaccid foot
5. locked: a bone that is unable to return to its natural position
6. motor nerves: the nervous tissue that carries messages to initiate muscular contraction
7. open fracture: a broken bone in which the bone ends erupt through the skin
8. osteoporosis: a softening of bones due to loss of calcium
9. position of function: the natural relaxed position of the hand or foot
10. range of motion: the movement of bone or limb allowed by a joint
11. sciatic nerve: the primary sensory and motor nerve of the legs
12. sensory nerve: the nervous tissue that carries impulses of feeling such as pressure or pain
13. spontaneous reduction: a bone that returns to its natural position without assistance
14. sprain: a stretch of a ligament or tendon beyond its range of motion resulting in tissue injury
15. traction: a steady inline pull

Matching:

1. f
2. g
3. a
4. c
5. b
6. e
7. d

True or False:

1. F
2. T
3. F
4. T
5. F
6. F
7. T
8. T
9. T
10. T
11. T
12. F
13. T
14. F
15. T

Fill in the Blank:

Next to most LONG BONES lies an artery, a NERVE, and a VEIN. Surrounding the bone are muscles, TENDONS, and soft tissues. Covering all of this is skin. If a broken bone end cuts an artery, there will be bleeding into the tissues, causing the area to become PAINFUL, SWOLLEN, and DEFORMED. Disruption of an artery can cause loss of PULSES distal to the injury.

If a sensory nerve is injured, the patient may complain of numbness or tingling, called PARESTHESIA. If the motor nerve has been injured, however, the EMT may see signs of weakness of movement or PARESIS. If there is no movement of the extremity or PARALYSIS, check the opposite extremity. Loss of movement on both sides should alert the EMT to possible SPINAL injury.

A grating sensation called CREPITUS can often be noted when the patient moves an injured extremity. This is caused by bone ends GRINDING against each other. It is not necessary for the EMT to elicit this. Sudden pain at the exact location of the injury is called POINT TENDERNESS.

During the general impression, the EMT may notice that the patient is protecting or self-splinting an injury. This is called GUARDING.

Listing:

1. Swelling
2. Pain
3. Deformity
4. Paralysis
5. Paresthesia
6. Pulselessness
7. Cyanosis
8. Crepitus
9. Point tenderness
10. Guarding/self-splinting

Reviewing:

1. Deformity
2. Contusion
3. Abrasion
4. Puncture
5. Burns
6. Tenderness
7. Laceration
8. Swelling

Short Answer:

1. Movement of the joints can cause movement of the bone ends, leading to pain and soft tissue damage.
2. Adjacent to the joints is an artery and a nerve. Attempting to realign the joint can cause them to become trapped, leading to further injury distal to the joint.
3. It may be impossible or impractical to transport the patient out of the wilderness. Because hospitals are closer in urban areas, this is unnecessary in most cases.

Critical Thinking 1:

1. Michael is awake, has an open airway, is breathing, and has adequate circulation at the moment. They know his arm hurts and he is self-splinting it.
2. Scene survey, general first impression, initial assessment, focused history, physical
3. Manually stabilize the arm. Check pulses, movement, and sensation. Apply a rigid splint, padding any voids. Keep the hand in a position of function. Secure the splint. Recheck pulses, movement, and sensation. Place the arm in a sling. Elevate it. Apply ice.
4. Yes, they would need to cover it with a dry, sterile dressing and splint in position found.
5. One attempt may be made to realign the ends and restore pulses. Consider contacting Medical Control.

Critical Thinking 2:

1. Most likely a patella dislocation
2. Agree

Chapter 26

Identification:

1. contraindication
2. bronchodilators
3. protocols
4. actions
5. dose
6. expiration date
7. off-line medical control
8. side effects
9. indication
10. standing orders

Identification:

__	Ventolin	X	pseudoephedrine	X	acetaminophen
X	ibuprofen	__	Sudafed	__	Motrin
__	Advil	X	albuterol	__	Tylenol

True or False:

1. F
2. T
3. F
4. T
5. F
6. F
7. T
8. F

Identification:

1. tablet
2. gel
3. suspension
4. nebulizer
5. gas

Naming:

1. IV
2. PO
3. SQ
4. IM
5. inhalation
6. SL

Listing:

1. right patient
2. medication
3. right route
4. right dose
5. right date

Fill in the Blank:

The EMT-B must ASSESS the patient and include physical and historical information on the patient care record. List the exact NAME of the drug, the DOSE, or how much was given, and the ROUTE, or the way it was given. Within 5 minutes of giving the medication, a REASSESSMENT of the patient should be done and findings from this should be included on the patient care record. Be sure to evaluate the signs or symptoms that led to the use of the medication originally.

Completion:

See text, and review Med Notes for each drug listed.

Critical Thinking 1:

1. albuterol
2. he had shortness of breath, a history of albuterol usage, wheezing in lungs
3. lung sounds, pt's ability to breathe

Critical Thinking 2:

1. EpiPen
2. wheezing, possible anaphylaxis
3. lung sounds, area affected with rash or swelling

Critical Thinking 3:

1. nitro
2. chest pressure, shortness of breath
3. chest pain, shortness of breath

Chapter 27

Word Scramble:

1. asthma
2. bronchospasm
3. crackles
4. croup
5. cyanosis
6. diffusion
7. dyspnea
8. epiglottitis
9. rhonchi
10. wheezing

Fill in the Blank:

1. accessory muscles of respiration
2. alveolar pulmonary gas exchange
3. cellular respiration
4. chronic obstructive pulmonary disease
5. congestive heart failure
6. hypoxic drive
7. pulmonary embolus
8. respiration, ventilation

Sorting:

Pediatric	**Adult**	**Both**
very flexible trachea	12-20 breaths per minute	wheezing
easily obstructed by slight swelling		
floppy large epiglottis		
tongue takes up most of mouth		
15–30 breaths per minute		

Matching:

1. c
2. d
3. e
4. g
5. f
6. b
7. a

Short Answer:

1. Pulmonary embolus: any from Table 27-1
2. COPD: cigarette smoking
3. Asthma: exercise, inhalants, cold, animal dander
4. Croup: child, upper respiratory infection
5. Epiglottitis: child

Completion:

Generic name	albuterol
Trade name	Ventolin, Proventil
Indication	Signs and symptoms of respiratory distress As prescribed by MD
Contraindication	Nonalert patient
Dose	Two puffs 1 minute apart
Route	Inhaled

Labeling

See Figure 27-1 in your text.

Short Answer:

1. Chronically high carbon dioxide levels cause the body to get used to the levels. The stimulus to breathe then becomes a low oxygen level.
2. Hypoperfusion is an acute event; the body does not have time to get used to it and switch over.

Critical Thinking 1:

1. Air passing through bronchioles narrowed by bronchospasm produces a musical or whistling sound called wheezing. In an asthma attack, some irritant causes the bronchospasm.
2. The reduction in wheezing meant that less and less air was moving through Kara's lower airways.
3. Diane must begin ventilation by bag-valve-mask. An ALS intercept should be requested if not already done so.

Critical Thinking 2:

1. Irritation of the larynx produces the characteristic barking cough.
2. Croup and epiglottis are often difficult to tell apart. The EMT should not examine Adam's mouth, as this could cause further swelling in the tissues and precipitate complete airway obstruction.

Critical Thinking 3:

1. Yes. Even though Mr. Williamson may be breathing based on hypoxic drive, he is currently having difficulty, and therefore oxygen should not be withheld.
2. Since cold air may further narrow his airways, the EMTs should be sure that he is adequately bundled up.

Chapter 28

Definitions:

1. angina
2. plaques
3. JVD
4. hypertension
5. thrombus
6. coronary
7. cardiogenic
8. myocardium
9. clot
10. tachycardia
11. diaphoretic
12. epigastrium
13. bradycardia
14. perfusion

Identification:
Modifiable: smoking, drugs, lack of exercise, diet
Nonmodifiable: sex, age, family history, hypertension, race, diabetes

Labeling:
See Figure 28-1 in your text.

Identification:
1. smoking
2. drugs
3. exercise
4. diet
5. sex
6. age
7. family history
8. hypertension
9. race
10. diabetes

True or False:
1. F
2. T
3. T
4. F
5. F
6. F
7. T
8. T
9. T
10. T

Ordering:
8 complete a focused physical exam
3 assess the airway
6 obtain baseline vital signs
7 get a SAMPLE history
1 survey the scene for safety
5 check circulation
2 note general impression
4 assess breathing adequacy

Short Answer:
1. Prompt recognition and treatment are the key to survival.
2. The heart muscle obtains its oxygen and nutrients from the coronary arteries.
3. The treatment for each is the same, so it is not essential for an EMT to make the distinction. The recognition of a possibility of an MI based on risk factors and history, plus appropriate treatment, is the important point.

Critical Thinking:
1. Past medical history using SAMPLE
   History of this illness using OPQRST
   Focused physical exam including assessment of jugular venous distention, breath sounds, vital signs, pulse oximetry, and pupils
2. They must reassess for relief from the medication and complete the components of the initial assessment and vital signs.
3. Be sure Mr. Stevens is lying down and has high-flow oxygen. They should have called for ALS intervention and can contact Medical Control for additional assistance.

Chapter 29

Definitions:
1. defibrillation: application of an electrical shock to the heart in ventricular fibrillation
2. dysrhythmia: any disruption of the normal sinus rhythm
3. electrocardiogram: the heart's electrical flow graphically displayed on paper or oscilloscope
4. automaticity: ability of the myocardium to self-pace
5. rhythm: regularly repeating ECG pattern
6. sudden cardiac death: unexpected cessation of heartbeat within 2 hours of the onset of chest pain
7. chain of survival: important steps that must be taken to improve cardiac arrest survival
8. public access defibrillation: public training in the use of an AED
9. artificial pacemaker: a man-made device that will create a spark, signaling the heart to beat
10. all clear command: an order that nothing should touch the patient

Labeling:
See Figure 29-7 in your text.

Identification:

A. asystole
B. sinus rhythm with PVCs
C. ventricular fibrillations
D. ventricular tachycardia

Ordering:

3 Open airway
1 BSI/scene safety
5 Check for carotid pulse
4 Observe for chest rise
2 Check responsiveness

Ordering:

3 Turn on AED and stop touching the patient
7 Reanalyze/reassess
4 Analyze rhythm
1 Assess patient
2 Apply patches/cable
5 Clear patient for shock
6 Press "shock" button

Identification

1. contraindication
2. contraindication
3. indication
4. contraindication
5. indication
6. contraindication
7. contraindication
8. contraindication
9. contraindication
10. indication

True or False:

1. F
2. T
3. F
4. F
5. T
6. F
7. T
8. T
9. T
10. T
11. T
12. F

Short Answer:

1. The pads will fit better. The shock will be adjusted down for the lower weight of a child. The sequence of shocks will reflect the pediatric algorithm.
2. The EMT will need to provide care and support to the survivors.

Critical Thinking 1:

1. One of the EMTs should obtain the AED, while the other assesses the patient and the performance of CPR.
2. Once the patient has been confirmed as unresponsive, pulseless, and apneic, the EMT should apply the patches, turn on the AED, clear the patient for analysis, analyze the rhythm, and if shock is advised, clear the patient and press the shock button. If no shock is advised they should continue CPR, prepare for transport, and call for ALS.
3. They should reassess the patient. If there is no pulse, continue CPR, prepare for transport, and contact ALS. If a pulse is present, they must assess adequacy of breathing, obtain vital signs, and prepare to transport.
4. The EMTs or paramedics should provide explanation and support to Mr. Roberts' family.

Critical Thinking 2:

1. The AED is to be used on patients who are unresponsive, pulseless, and apneic. The patient does not meet these criteria.
2. The EMT supervisor should tell Bev and Joe that it would be better if they didn't apply the patches just yet. He could offer to assist with further care and packaging. After the call is complete, the supervisor will need to review the standards of AED use with Bev and Joe. The EMTs may need to complete an AED refresher course of study.

Chapter 30

Matching:

1. n
2. l
3. k
4. h
5. g
6. e
7. j
8. f
9. c
10. b
11. o
12. m
13. a
14. d
15. i

Correcting:

1. A person experiencing a change in behavior that may be due to illness or injury is having a behavioral crisis.
2. A failure to remember what just happened is called amnesia.
3. Hypoglycemia is a lack of sugar in the blood.
4. Diabetes mellitus occurs when the pancreas fails to produce sufficient insulin.
5. Excessive urination is called polyuria.
6. The development of hypoglycemia is a short-term event, often occuring over minutes to hours.
7. When the body cannot use sugar for energy, it uses fat instead.
8. Kussmaul's respirations are fast and deep.
9. Insulin shock results from low sugar in the blood.
10. A patient experiencing a low blood sugar will have cool, moist skin.
11. The cause of epilepsy is not well defined.
12. In a seizure affecting the whole brain, the full body is affected.
13. An aura is an odor or flash of light or sound that precedes certain seizures.
14. The postictal phase of a seizure occurs after the body has seized.
15. Managing a seizing patient includes isolating the body from hazards.

Short Answer:

1. The brain malfunctions when glucose is not available because it is the primary source of energy for the body.
2. A person can still produce insulin; however, she may not produce enough to balance her diet.
3. Epilepsy is a disease of the electrical conduction throughout the brain. Seizures can also be caused by trauma or illnesses.
4. Patients can have a partial seizure and still remain standing. It would appear that they were "daydreaming" or lost the ability to speak.

Critical Thinking 1:

1. It may have been caused by low blood sugar.
2. They should follow the ABCs and call for ALS.
3. Oral glucose is contraindicated, because the patient is unconscious and unresponsive.

Critical Thinking 2:

1. Head trauma from a fall may have caused this condition.
2. The EMTs should isolate the patient from any potential hazards and then attempt to protect and stabilize the head, neck, and spine.
3. C-spine precautions and ABC management should be the EMTs' first priority.
4. No, because the patient is not conscious.
5. Yes, oxygen is indicated, because the child is unconscious.

Chapter 31

Matching:

1. d
2. e
3. a
4. c
5. b

Definitions:

1. stroke: permanent brain injury caused by an interruption in blood flow
2. hemorrhagic stroke: blood flow is interrupted due to a rupture of one of the cerebral vessels
3. ischemic stroke: blood flow is interrupted due to a thrombus or embolus blocking a cerebral vessel
4. cerebrovascular accident (CVA): the medical name for a stroke
5. transient ischemic attack (TIA): a temporary interruption in blood flow
6. embolus: a clot that travels
7. thrombus: a blood clot

Labeling:

See Figure 31-3 of your text.

Listing:

Component	Normal	Abnormal	Way to assess
Facial droop	Both sides of the face move equally	One side doesn't move	Ask patient to smile
Arm drift	Both arms move equally or not at all	One arm drifts	Ask patient to close eyes and hold arms out in front
Speech	Uses correct words without slurring	Slurred or incorrect words	Ask patient to repeat a sentence

Identification:

1. hypoglycemia
2. Bell's palsy
3. traumatic brain injury
4. seizure
5. migraine
6. drug toxicity

Short Answer:

1. Management of life threats to the ABCs with timely transport

Critical Thinking 1:

1. stroke, transient ischemic attack, hypoglycemia, Bell's palsy, traumatic brain injury, seizure, migraine, drug toxicity
2. Manage Mr. Mantelli's airway, breathing, and circulation, and transport him to the appropriate hospital as quickly as possible, They should call for advanced life support assistance and perhaps consider helicopter transport. They should notify the hospital of Mr. Mantelli's symptoms and current condition.
3. Debra and Brian should tell Mrs. Mantelli that her husband's symptoms could be caused by a specific type of headache, changes in his blood sugar, or a stroke. They should indicate that she did the right thing by calling EMS and that her husband needs to be transported to the hospital. They should keep her informed of Mr. Mantelli's condition and their care.

Critical Thinking 2:

1. stroke, transient ischemic attack, hypoglycemia, Bell's palsy, traumatic brain injury, seizure, migraine, drug toxicity
2. In addition to an initial exam, focused history, and physical and vital signs, the EMTs should have the patient complete the Cincinnati Stroke Scale. They should complete ongoing exams as frequently as indicated.
3. Manage his airway, breathing, and circulation, and transport him to the appropriate hospital as quickly as possible, They should call for advanced life support assistance and perhaps consider helicopter transport. They should notify the hospital of the patient's symptoms and current condition.
4. The EMTs appropriately treated this patient for the worse possible condition, the stroke.

Chapter 32

Matching:

1. i
2. g
3. d
4. j
5. h
6. f
7. o
8. c
9. b
10. a

Identification:

1. tactile
2. command
3. visual
4. auditory
5. auditory
6. command
7. tactile
8. visual

Identification:

1. extremity
2. extremity
3. total body
4. papoose
5. takedown
6. positional asphyxia
7. four people
8. show of force
9. medically necessary

Sorting:

1. ___ A young mother is crying after the death of her infant.
2. X A teenager is threatening to shoot himself after getting a bad grade.
Request police assistance for safety. Once the scene is safe, be supportive but decisive.
3. X A young man is crying loudly after he dropped his soda.
One EMT should perform the initial assessment and develop the history. He should speak slowly and clearly, be honest, and be supportive but decisive.
4. ___ A middle-aged woman is upset that she is having breathing difficulties.
5. ___ An elderly man is afraid that he will die if he enters a hospital.
6. X A young man threatens to kill all people who wear uniforms.
Request police for safety. Have nonuniformed personnel approach the patient when it is safe to do so. One EMT should perform the initial assessment and develop the history. He should speak slowly and clearly, be honest, and be supportive but decisive.
7. ___ A middle-aged man expresses anger that his wife just died.
8. ___ A newly arrived immigrant cannot follow your directions.
9. ___ A young man is upset after the saw he was using sliced his hand.
10. X A teenaged girl states she is going to stab all the snakes in the room.
Request police for safety. Be sure the girl is unarmed. One EMT should perform the initial assessment and develop the history. He should speak slowly and clearly, be honest, and not attempt to confirm or deny any hallucination.

True or False:

1. F
2. T
3. T
4. F
5. T
6. T
7. T
8. F
9. T
10. F

Short Answer:

1. This patient is assumed to not be in a frame of mind where she is capable of making decisions regarding her health.
2. Four people are recommended, in order to maintain the safety of the crew.
3. The EMT should sit at the head of the patient, where he can manage the ABCs and speak directly to the patient.
4. When a patient is restrained, pulses, movement, and sensation should be checked every 5–10 minutes.

Critical Thinking 1:

1. Yes, it is a situation in which the man's behavior is unacceptable to himself, family, or the community.
2. Yes, based on the medic alert bracelet, it is very probable that the behavior is being caused by a malfunction of the brain due to incorrect sugar levels.
3. They should try to assist the man into the ambulance so that he is not being viewed by onlookers. They should call for ALS, as it is possible that the man will be unable to follow directions to take sugar, or that he will be unable to control his airway. They should request the police unit to try to contact the man's family.

Critical Thinking 2:

1. Yes, the patient is exhibiting behavior that is intolerable to self, family, or community.
2. The EMTs must be nonjudgmental and nonconfrontational, while ensuring they are able to withdraw as necessary. They should choose or alter their approach to avoid offending the patient.
3. Janie must remember that the patient is ill and comments made are under duress. She should not take the comments personally.
4. She should maintain a professional attitude, clearly identify herself, and state her intentions clearly.
5. Only one EMT should speak to the patient. This allows trust to be built and also decreases the possibilty of confusion.

Chapter 33

Matching:

1. c
2. f
3. h
4. i
5. a
6. k
7. l
8. e
9. b
10. d
11. g
12. j

Definitions:

1. hematochezia: passage of bright red blood from the rectum
2. hemetemesis: vomitus that mostly consists of blood
3. jaundice: a yellow discoloration of the skin caused by excess bilirubin in the blood
4. melena: tarry dark stool caused by bleeding in the upper gastrointestinal tract

Listing:

1. stomach, small intestine, large intestine, pancreas, liver, gallbladder
2. kidney, ureters, bladder
3. spleen, blood vessels

Short Answer:

Altered glucose/insulin metabolism, loss of fluids, bleeding

Critical Thinking:

1. A kidney stone
2. They should prepare Mr. Smythe for immediate transport, assist him into a position of comfort as much as is possible, continue the oxygen therapy, and call for advanced life support assistance.
3. The paramedic is likely to provide fluids by IV and give medications for pain control and vomiting.

Chapter 34

Matching:

1. i
2. l
3. o
4. a
5. h
6. k
7. m
8. b
9. c
10. n
11. d
12. j
13. e
14. g
15. f

Sorting:

	Radiation	Convection	Conduction	Evaporation
Removing your sweater in a cool room	X			
Sitting on cold rocks			X	
Breathing				X
Sitting in front of a fan		X		
Turning on the air conditioner in the house	X			
Entering a meat cooler	X			
Sweating				X
Swimming in a cold lake			X	
Standing in the wind		X		
Lying on a waterbed heated to 70°F			X	

Identification:

X diabetes mellitus
__ adolescent
X heart disease
X multiple medications
__ isolated broken wrist
X generalized infection
X burns
__ sprained ankle
X thyroid condition
X head injury
X shock
__ infected tooth
X spinal cord injury

Treatments:

Local cold injuries: remove patient from cold or wet environment, remove cold or wet clothing, rewarm injured part

Hypothermia: assess body temperature; remove patient from cold environment; remove cold, wet clothing; cover with warm blankets; administer oxygen (preferably warmed and humidified), prevent further heat loss

Heat cramps: remove patient from hot environment, gently massage painful area, rehydrate orally with water or electrolyte solution

Heat exhaustion: remove patient from hot environment, remove excess clothing, rehydrate orally with water or electrolyte solutions, call for ALS

Heat stroke: remove the patient from hot environment, provide aggressive cooling measures, monitor ABCs, administer oxygen, transport, call for ALS

Snake bites: keep patient calm, immobilize extremity, keep below level of heart, transport to hospital, consider ALS intercept

Sorting:

1. X poor coordination
2. __ flushing
3. __ nausea
4. X slurred speech
5. X poor judgment
6. X slow pulse
7. X pale skin
8. __ stomach cramps
9. X mood changes
10. X decreased sensation
11. __ muscle cramps
12. __ itching

Identification:

1. active
2. passive
3. active
4. passive
5. passive
6. active
7. active
8. passive

Ordering:

3 row
1 reach
4 go
2 throw

Listing:

descent: squeeze (air-filled spaces like sinus)
ascent: decompression sickness, pulmonary overpressurization, air embolism

Fill in the Blank:

Lightning strikes are divided into MINOR and SEVERE injuries. With lesser injuries, the common symptoms include CONFUSION, AMNESIA, and short-term memory difficulties. A large percentage of people suffer ruptured EARDRUMS. They may also suffer BLUNT trauma. The EMT should IMMOBILIZE the patient to prevent any further injuries.

In other people, the electricity produces a shock that stops CARDIAC electrical activity and a full arrest occurs. Even if the heart resumes function, the BRAIN may continue to malfunction, preventing RESPIRATORY effort and resulting in hypoxia. The first priority in the management of a victim of a lightning strike is SCENE SAFETY.

Short Answer:

1. Any two: convection, conduction, radiation, or evaporation
2. Routine cellular metabolism and muscle contraction are internal ways for the body to gain heat. An external source is for the body to absorb heat from a warmer environment.
3. Vasoconstriction, piloerection
4. The old or very young may be unable to remove themselves from the environment, or put on or remove clothing. They have a variation in amount of insulation.
5. Afterdrop results from peripheral vasodilation resulting from application of warm items to the skin. The cold blood caught out in the periphery is then sent back to the core of the body, resulting in a temperature drop.
6. Neurological damage, respiratory difficulties.
7. Any injury resulting during a dive can leave the patient at risk for a drowning or near-drowning episode.
8. Mountain sickness results from a decreased amount of oxygen in the air. The patient has not acclimated to this decreased oxygen and therefore suffers symptoms of hypoxia. Oxygen is used to both treat the illness and assist in acclimating to the environment.

Critical Thinking 1:

1. Lightning strike
2. Scene safety
3. If the man on the ground is in cardiac arrest, they should care for him first.
4. Trauma, including spinal injuries due to falls

Critical Thinking 2:

1. They know that the event took place within the past 24 hours, as the mailman had noticed that she was fine yesterday.
2. They should provide general hypothermia management.

Critical Thinking 3:

1. He was likely bitten by a black widow spider.
2. Bandage the site of the bite and provide supportive care.
3. Yes, some black widow bites can result in death. George should receive a complete evaluation at the hospital.

Chapter 35

Matching:

1. d
2. f
3. j
4. g
5. a
6. h
7. i
8. b
9. c
10. e

Definitions:

1. allergic reaction: an expected activation of the immune system upon an exposure to a particular substance
2. epinephrine: an injectable medication that dilates the bronchioles and constricts the blood vessels
3. ingestion: taken in orally
4. inhalation: taken in through the respiratory tract
5. injected: taken in through a hole made in the skin
6. absorbed: taken in through intact skin
7. poisoning: exposure to a substance that results in illness

Identification:

1. injected
2. injected
3. ingested or absorbed
4. inhaled
5. inhaled
6. absorbed or inhaled
7. inhaled or absorbed
8. absorbed
9. ingested
10. inhaled

True or False:

1. T
2. F
3. F
4. F
5. T
6. T
7. F

Completion:

Generic name	activated charcoal
Trade name	Actidose, SuperChar
Indication	recent ingestion of susceptible poison
Contraindication	inability to control airway or swallow
Dose	1 gram/kg (50–100 g adults)
Route	orally

Completion:

Generic name	Epinephrine
Trade name	EpiPen
Indication	life-threatening allergic reaction
Contraindication	none as long as indicated
Dose	0.3–0.5 mg adults (contents of injector)
Route	intramuscular

Short Answer:

1. Mild = Localized swelling   Severe = More generalized swelling
2. Respiratory signs including throat tightness, shortness of breath, cough, wheezing, stridor, hoarseness, tachypnea
   Cardiovascular signs including tachycardia, hypotension, dizziness, hypoperfusion
   Sense of impending doom
   Decreasing mental status, increasing difficulty breathing, decreasing blood pressure

Critical Thinking 1:

1. Absorption through his hands.
2. He should lie down or sit down, wash or wipe the remainder of the paste off his skin, and be monitored by an EMT.

Critical Thinking 2:

1. Injected with fluid from the wasps.
2. She should be given high-flow oxygen, ALS should be called, and EpiPen administration could be considered if the indications for such are present.

Critical Thinking 3:

1. Inhalation of toxic gas
2. Once correctly trained personnel have removed Aimee from the apartment, she should be given high-flow oxygen, ventilated if necessary, and ALS should be called.

Chapter 36

True or False:

1. F
2. T
3. F
4. F

5. F
6. T
7. F
8. T
9. T
10. T

Identification:

1. Abortion
2. Eclampsia
3. Placenta previa
4. Supine hypotensive syndrome
5. Appendicitis
6. Miscarriage
7. Ectopic pregnancy
8. Placental abruption

Fill in the Blank:

Pregnancy changes the way the body takes care of itself. The pregnant woman's heart is normally HIGHER than the nonpregnant woman's, and her blood pressure is usually LOWER. The EMT should remember that the pregnant woman has manufactured approximately 30% more blood than usual, and so a significant blood loss can occur before there is a change in VITAL SIGNS.

The EMT must remember that in managing any trauma in pregnancy, she must concentrate on saving the MOTHER.

Short Answer:

1. Skin signs; the normal vital signs have been changed by the process of pregnancy. The mother in shock will shunt blood away from the fetus and also away from the skin. The EMT can make observations about the skin.
2. Falls, blunt trauma in MVC, intentional violence
3. The mother's center of gravity changes, placing her at greater risk of losing her balance. In MVC, the abdomen is likely to strike the steering wheel or dash first. Pregnancy causes many emotions, not only in the woman but also her partner, placing her at risk for domestic violence.

Critical Thinking:

1. Scene safety/size-up, general first impression, initial assessment, focused history and physical, vital signs. Pay attention to the skin signs.
2. Placenta previa
3. They should manage her in the same way regardless of the cause. Place her supine and turned to her left side. Give high-flow oxygen. Call for ALS if not done already. Transport to an appropriate facility. Continue with ongoing assessments.

Chapter 37

Word Scramble:

1. effacement
2. labor
3. multiparous
4. primiparous
5. crowning
6. gravida
7. para
8. molding
9. meconium

Definitions:

1. amniotic sac: the membranous sac that surrounds the fetus in the uterus
2. cervical dilation: progressive opening of the cervix that occurs as the fetal head descends into the pelvis
3. bloody show: expulsion of a small amount of bloody mucus from the cervix as it begins to thin
4. Braxton Hicks contractions: random contractions that occur in the third trimester; also known as false labor
5. cardinal movements of labor: series of natural movements the infant makes upon descent through the birth canal
6. prolapsed umbilical cord: presentation of the umbilical cord before the infant; results in compression of the cord
7. breech presentation: presentation of foot or buttocks first instead of the infant's head
8. premature delivery: a delivery that occurs before the 37th week of the pregnancy

Sorting:

First stage	**Second stage**	**Third stage**
effacement	delivery of the infant	delivery of the placenta
rupture of amniotic sac	infant's head pushing on rectum	gushing of blood, approximately 250–500 cc
full cervical dilation	crowning	

Identification:

X Due date
__ Blood pressure
X Any complications during the pregnancy
__ Crowning
X Prenatal care
__ Any fluids from the vagina
X Time when contractions started
__ BSI
__ Maternal weight
X How long each contraction lasts
X Gravida
X Parity

Sorting:

Field delivery
crowning
multiparous, contractions 2 minutes apart
need to move bowels
need to push
increased vaginal pressure

Transport
primiparous, contractions 10 minutes apart
irregular contractions
primiparous, regular contractions, no observation of fetal head

Listing:

1. Surgical scissors are used to cut the cord.
2. Clamps are used to clamp the cord in two places.
3. Bulb syringe is used to suction the mouth and nose.
4. Towels are used to dry the infant.
5. Gauze sponges are used to wipe blood.
6. BSI is necessary for self-protection. There are many fluids during a delivery.
7. The blanket is to keep the infant warm.
8. A plastic bag is used to transport the placenta to the hospital.

Ordering:

9 Deliver placenta
2 Position the mother
3 Gentle pressure on the infant's head during crowning
4 Check for cord around the neck
10 Record time and place of delivery
5 Suction mouth and then nose of infant
1 BSI
7 Clamp cord when pulsations have stopped
8 Dry infant and wrap
6 Support the infant's weight during delivery
11 Transport mother, infant, and placenta to hospital

Critical Thinking:

1. See Table 37-2 in your text.
2. The EMTs need to tell Grace that delivery is imminent, and that they will assist her in delivering her infant at home. They need to be supportive.
3. Yes, since Grace has not had prenatal care and her infant is arriving early (premature), the EMTs would be wise to obtain any needed advice.
4. Twins
5. The EMTs need to prepare for the second delivery by obtaining a second OB kit and by calling for additional personnel.

Chapter 38

True or False:

1. F
2. T
3. F
4. F
5. F
6. T
7. F
8. F
9. F
10. T

Sorting:

1. __ suckling
2. X placing the newborn on a table (place on a blanket or towel)
3. __ positioning the newborn on mother's abdomen

4. X leaving baby's head uncovered to monitor fontanelles (dry and cover the head)
5. X letting infant stay in amniotic fluid (dry the infant)
6. __ swaddling

Ordering:

5 ALS drugs
2 Blow-by oxygen
4 Chest compressions
1 Drying, warming, and positioning
3 BVM

Fill in the Blank:

Measuring heart rate, respiratory effort, muscle tone, responses, and color in the newborn is determined through the use of the APGAR score. It is completed at 1 and 5 minutes after birth. The EMT must also assess the newborn's airway. Place the newborn supine and slightly head down. Use a BULB SYRINGE to clear the newborn's NOSTRILS. The newborn is an obligate NOSE breather. Respirations must be adequate. Crying is a good sign. Even though respirations are adequate, the newborn may have blue hands and feet. This is called ACROCYANOSIS. A heart rate of less than 60 beats per minute means that the EMT must begin chest compressions. Once the initial assessment and Apgar is completed, begin a FOCUSED medical assessment. Sometimes the infant's head may appear misshapen. This results from the birth and is called MOLDING. The head shape will return to normal. The EMT must assess the UMBILICAL cord, which should appear bluish white. The EMT must take care to appear professional and nonjudgmental, as new parents "read" the expressions and behaviors of the caregivers.

Calculation:

1. 9
2. 2
3. 7
4. 1
5. 10

Short Answer:

1. The infant produces a lot of mucus during his first few minutes to hours, and the infant is an obligate nose breather.
2. Nasal flaring, bradycardia, retractions, seesaw respirations, grunting

Critical Thinking:

1. 1
2. ABCs, utilizing the inverted pyramid of newborn care
3. Honesty, complete explanation of all care

Chapter 39

Word Scramble:

1. croup
2. asthma
3. meningitis
4. epiglottitis
5. debriefing
6. retractions
7. febrile

Completion:

See Table 39-1 of your text.

True or False:

1. T
2. F
3. F
4. T
5. T
6. T
7. T
8. F
9. T
10. F
11. T
12. F
13. F
14. T
15. T

Matching:

1. i
2. h
3. f
4. g
5. b
6. c
7. d
8. j
9. e
10. a

Correcting:

1. Unknown
2. 1 week and 1 year
3. Sleeping
4. Lower
5. Remove the word "not"
6. Cannot
7. During the resuscitation
8. Remove the word "not"

Short Answer:

1. Aspiration of a foreign body
2. The child's airway is smaller and more likely to become obstructed by swelling.
3. No, the two illnesses are treated the same way in the field.
4. Signs of hypoperfusion include: increased heart rate, pale skin color, delayed capillary refill, nausea, a decreased urinary output, changes in the child's level of consciousness, and an eventual drop in blood pressure.

Critical Thinking 1:

1. Yes, there are signs that this child has a severe illness called meningitis.
2. The EMTs should wear gloves and a mask.
3. The EMTs need to provide explanations of what they are doing, and give caring support to Mrs. Smythe.

Critical Thinking 2:

1. No
2. The child has a good airway, as evidenced by his cough and yelling.

Chapter 40

Fill in the Blank:

1. mandated reporter
2. mechanical ventilator
3. cerebrospinal fluid shunt
4. tracheostomy
5. child abuse
6. feeding tube
7. tracheostomy tube
8. central venous catheter

Identification:

Toddler	motor vehicle collisions pools and buckets scalding household cleaners/pills
School-aged	motor vehicle collisions bikes intentional fires
Adolescent	motor vehicle collisions suicide/homicide drug ingestion/overdose

Assessments:

General impression: Compare this child's actions to those of a noninjured child. Any answers indicating a deviation from age norms are acceptable.
Mental status: inactive, lack of attention to environment, dull eyes, self-absorbed
Airway: breathing through open mouth (air hunger)
Breathing: seesaw respirations, retractions
Circulation: pale, cool, tachycardic, delayed capillary refill

Short Answer:

1. A child's head is larger, proportionally. This makes him more top heavy and more prone to head injuries.
2. Comfort and cooperation from a child in more familiar surroundings, or convenience of move from vehicle to ambulance
3. Swelling in the airway, inhalations of toxins from the fire, hypothermia
4. Pattern of injury does not match reported mechanism of injury, several injuries in various stages of healing, responding to same address repeatedly for injuries. The EMT should document accurately and without making judgments. The EMT should also report her observations to the physician.
5. Children with special needs may have vital signs and responses that are not usual for most children but are normal for that child. Caregivers usually have a clear understanding of baseline information.

Identification:

1. trauma center
2. local hospital
3. local hospital
4. trauma center
5. trauma center
6. trauma center
7. trauma center
8. trauma center
9. local hospital
10. trauma center

Chapter 41

Matching:

1. f
2. a
3. e
4. b
5. c
6. d

Identification:

1. Visual acuity declines
2. Progressive decline in hearing
3. Stiffening of blood vessels
   Buildup of fatty deposits in blood vessels
   Decrease in exercise tolerance
   Diminished effectiveness of heart as a pump
4. Decreased elasticity of chest wall and lung tissue, indicating a decrease in lung volume
   Inefficiency of cilia and cough mechanism
   Decreased oxygen uptake
5. Loss of teeth
   Decreased motility of GI tract, with inefficient absorption of nutrients
6. Decline in kidney function
   Loss of bladder tone and capacity
7. Loss of calcium from bone
   Decreased flexibility in joints
8. Loss of fat beneath the skin
   Decreased effectiveness of sweat glands

Fill in the Blank:

In the over 65 year-old population, TRAUMA is the fifth leading cause of death. FALLS account for the most significant injuries in the adult. In obtaining a history, it is important for the EMT to question EVENTS that occurred before any falls. Even minor HEAD trauma can lead to significant injury. Subtle symptoms such as CONFUSION or HEADACHE can occur days to weeks after the injury.

More than half of all MYOCARDIAL INFARCTIONS (MI) occur in elderly patients. Their symptoms may be unusual, including SHORTNESS of BREATH, NAUSEA, DIZZINESS, WEAKNESS OR SWEATING even without chest pain. Abdominal pain in an elderly patient can mean a SERIOUS CONDITION. Many elderly patients with severe infection do not have a FEVER.

Short Answer:

1. Level of consciousness declines in delirium; it remains normal in dementia.
2. Delirium is usually caused by an acute medical condition that can be treated and reversed.

Critical Thinking:

1. Dementia, likely Alzheimer's disease
2. They must consider vascular problems, subdural hemorrhage or other trauma, infections, alcohol use or drug intoxication, and depression.
3. No, patients with Alzheimer's disease may develop a worsening of their symptoms when other medical conditions are present.
4. Lisa and Tony should perform a complete patient assessment, including initial assessment, focused history, and physical, as well as obtain a complete history from the son. It may be advisable to obtain information from the Adult Day Service Center also.
5. The son needs emotional support; it is often difficult to provide care for elderly parents. He also needs a step-by-step explanation of the reasons for the exam and history gathering.
6. Optimal care would include placing the woman on the stretcher in a comfortable position, obtaining a complete set of vital signs, respectfully obtaining the physical exam, and transporting the woman to a hospital. Of key importance is respect and compassion for the woman and her family.

Chapter 42

Definitions:

1. advance directive: a method to make a patient's wishes about resuscitation known to family and health care providers
2. DNR order: a physician's order to not start CPR or revive a patient in cardiac arrest
3. health care proxy: a person chosen to make medical decisions on behalf of another
4. living will: legal documents directing a patient's care if he becomes unable to do so
5. power of attorney: a designated person to make decisions for another

True or False:

1. F
2. F
3. T
4. T
5. T
6. F
7. F
8. T
9. T
10. T

Short Answer:

1. Consent and the right to withhold consent
2. The first two are legal documents requiring attorney involvement, while the second two require physician involvement.

Critical Thinking 1:

1. The EMTs need to assess the patient and determine if she is apneic and pulseless. If their system allows acceptance of a DNR, then they should honor the DNR. If they cannot honor it, they must give clear explanation to the family. Any questions can be directed to the Medical Control physician.
2. Regardless of the outcome, the granddaughter needs support and the opportunity to express her grief.

Critical Thinking 2:

1. Based on the unclear situation, the EMTs should begin resuscitation under the doctrine of implied consent. Questions can be directed to the Medical Control physician.

Chapter 43

Matching:

1. k
2. h
3. f
4. l
5. a
6. n
7. b
8. m
9. d
10. c
11. e
12. o
13. g
14. j
15. i

Definitions:

1. controlled intersection: an intersection with a traffic control device
2. yelp: a sharp, quick chirping type siren sound
3. LZ officer: designated person at scene of an incident who is responsible for choosing a landing zone and ensuring its safety
4. covering the brake: placing one foot over the brake in anticipation of stopping
5. surrounding area: space above and around the helicopter touchdown site
6. emergency ambulances: vehicles specifically designed for patient transportation
7. four-second rule: the amount of time separating the emergency vehicle from the one in front of it; usually calculated against a fixed object such as a pole or parked car
8. emergency services vehicle: a vehicle used by either fire, police, or EMS department
9. touchdown area: area within the landing zone where a helicopter will actually land
10. wail: a steady siren sound that ascends and then descends in pitch

Listing:

1. trained
2. rested
3. physically prepared
4. mentally prepared

Listing:

1. required items are where they belong
2. items function
3. electrical equipment is charged
4. batteries are charged
5. oxygen is available, portable tanks are filled and functional
6. equipment is clean

Listing:

See Table 43-5 in your text.

Listing:

See Table 43-5 in your text.

Descriptions:

1. Alarm and alert: communications center notified of event; may EMD[QA] the call
2. Initial information: communication specialist will give EMT sufficient information to find the call, know what equipment might be necessary, and be aware of any special concerns such as access
3. Departure: locate call on map, disconnect shoreline, crew members wear seat belts
4. Driving: using appropriate response mode, red lights and sirens for high priority, normal speed and following all traffic laws for low priority
5. Arrival: position ambulance, notify communications
6. On-scene actions: keep communications aware; nature of incident, number of patients, added resources, patient assessment and care, packaging and movement of patient to ambulance
7. Transport to facility: decision as to how and what priority, secure patient and crew in vehicle
8. Arrival at facility: notify communications, position ambulance
9. Transfer of care: move patient from ambulance cot to facility stretcher, raise siderails, lock wheels, secure equipment such as IV lines or oxygen, give complete verbal report, give patient belongings to receiving staff, provide written documentation
10. Preparation for next call: clean, decontaminate and restock, ensure adequate fuel

Short Answer:

ƎƆИA⅃UꓭMA is "ambulance" spelled backwards and reversed.

Critical Thinking 1:

1. Based on mechanism of injury, extent of injury, and a lengthy extrication; the helicopter appears to be a good choice for transport.
2. Choose a landing zone as close to scene as is safely possible
   Have a space of 75–100 square feet
   Have a slope of less than 10 degrees
   Surrounding area free of obstacles
   Mark the landing zone

Observe the descent of the helicopter. Wave pilot off if landing becomes unsafe
Remain in sight of the pilot. Do not permit anyone to approach until signaled by the pilot. Approach should be from the front at 12 o'clock position.

Critical Thinking 2:

1. Heavy traffic, distance, urban setting, rain, darkness, their physical condition, priority
2. priority—use caution, exercise due regard, use calming techniques

Other answers may be appropriate to a specific region of the country.

Chapter 44

Definitions:

1. chain of command: a system where every person has a superior, and that superior then reports to the Incident Commander
2. command post: area where fire, EMS, and police run a unified command of the incident
3. decontamination corridor: area that bridges the hot and cold zones; hazardous materials are cleaned off personnel here
4. hot zone: immediate area of a Hazmat spill; obvious risk to personnel at this area
5. Material Safety Data Sheets (MSDS): listing of health and safety information on various substances
6. multiple casualty incident (MCI): an event where the number of patients outweigh the number of EMTs
7. NFPA 704 symbol: a diamond-shaped warning sign, with four or more smaller diamonds inside of the larger one
8. START triage system: a popular triage system, standing for "simple triage and rapid treatment"
9. placard: system of symbols, indicating a certain class of hazardous material
10. triage: prioritizing patients based upon urgency

Matching:

1. c
2. f
3. i
4. e
5. g
6. j
7. h
8. d
9. b
10. a

Identification:

1. yellow
2. green
3. red
4. green
5. yellow
6. black
7. red
8. red
9. yellow
10. black

Ordering:

6 Warm zone is established with a decontamination corridor
5 Hot zone is established
4 Hazmat team is dispatched
1 The first unit arrives at the scene of a rolled over tanker truck
7 Patients are extracted from the tanker
8 Patients are decontaminated
9 Patients are treated
2 EMS command is established
10 Patients are transported
3 Ambulance is staged in the cold zone

Fill in the Blank:
Refer to Figure 44-22 in your text for the completed START triage algorithm.

Research:

1. camphor
2. gasoline
3. helium
4. potassium cyanide
5. propyl alcohol, normal
6. 1415
7. 1514
8. 1692
9. 1072
10. 2802

11. Move victim to fresh air
    Call 9-1-1
    Apply artificial respiration if not breathing. DO NOT use mouth to mouth if victim has ingested the substance
    Administer oxygen
    Remove and isolate clothing
    Flush skin or eyes for 20 minutes
    Avoid spreading material
    Keep victim quiet and warm
    Note effects may be delayed
    Ensure all medical personnel are aware of the substance involved and take steps to protect self

Short Answer:
The mnemonic SIN stands for safety, isolation, no entry.

Critical Thinking 1:
1. Establish command and designate a command post
   Declare an emergency and implement any preplans
   Appoint officers
   Coordinate with other emergency agencies
   Relinquish command when appropriately relieved
2. Safety officer, staging, triage, treatment, and transportation
3. Appoint a public information officer

Critical Thinking 2:
1. *Emergency Response Guidebook* by placard
   CHEMTREC
   Shipping papers
   (less specific) placard symbols and colors
2. Call for resources and establish a perimeter
3. Hot zone: special units
   Cold zone: EMS and other emergency workers

Chapter 45

Matching:
1. f
2. d
3. g
4. i
5. h
6. a
7. b
8. e
9. j
10. c

Identification:
1. V
2. V
3. V
4. V
5. W
6. W
7. V
8. W
9. W
10. B

Identification:
1. Personal protective equipment
2. Ear plugs
3. Boots and gloves
4. Goggles
5. Safety vest
6. Turnout coat
7. Helmet

Short Answer:

1. Swift water:
   EMS plays primarily a supporting role
   Locate the victim
   Attempt a shore-based rescue (reach, throw), if realistic
   Establish a base for the dive team
   Always wear a PFD if you are near the water
   Flat water:
   Reach
   Throw
   Row
   Then go if no other alternative means of rescue is avaliable
   Always wear a PFD
2. Phases of a rescue include: command, size-up, access and rescue, treatment, and transport
3. Helmet, eye protection, rip-resistant coat, heavy-duty work gloves

Critical Thinking 1:

1. Heavy rescue
2. Any three might include traffic, unstable tractor with load of sand, cab over bridge

Critical Thinking 2:

1. Shore rescue
2. Any three might include water itself, debris in the water, fuel in the water

Critical Thinking 3:

1. Confined space
2. Any three might include uneven terrain; falling rocks; lack of lighting, water, cool temperatures

Chapter 46

True or False:

1. F
2. F
3. F
4. F
5. T
6. F
7. T
8. T
9. F
10. T

Identification:

1	Transportation	Department of Transportation
2.	Communication	National Communications System
3.	Public Works	Department of Defense
4.	Firefighting	U.S. Department of Agriculture
5.	Information/Planning	Federal Emergency Management Agency
6.	Mass Care	American Red Cross
7.	Resource Support	Government Supply Agency
8.	Health and Medical Services	U.S. Department of Health and Human Resources
9.	Urban Search and Rescue	Federal Emergency Management Agency
10.	Hazardous Materials	U.S. Environmental Protection Agency
11.	Food	U.S. Department of Agriculture
12.	Energy	U.S. Department of Energy

Matching:

1. d
2. e
3. b
4. c
5. a

Short Answer:

1. T Wear firefighter protective gear.
2. R Avoid lengthy exposure, move away from the incident, use barriers such as concrete abutments.
3. A Stage upwind.
4. C Wait for the patient to be decontaminated.
5. E Use personal protective equipment.
6. M Consider use of ballistic protection such as a vest.

Critical Thinking:

1. It is possibly a domestic terrorist incident due to a targeted group and an unexplained explosion.
2. Numerous answers are acceptable, including secondary devices, radiation or biologic exposure, and snipers nearby.
3. No, due to the hazards listed above, Corey and Tom should call for appropriate resources.
4. Contamination means being physically covered with nuclear material and that material continues to emit radiation. Irradiated means a person was exposed and injured from nuclear material but does not pose a further threat to self or others.
5. Time, distance, and shielding

Chapter 47

Missing Letters:

farm chemicals
gr**a**in bins
tractor **r**ollover
SLUDGE**M**

b**e**lts
peri**m**eter
PP**E**
operator er**r**or
au**g**er
pull**e**ys
nitrogen dioxide
cows
act**i**on circle
manur**e** storage
hor**s**es

Definitions:

1. rollover protective structures: protective bars or canopies that prevent the operator from being crushed
2. power take-off: a spinning shaft that transfers the tractor engine's power to another piece of farm equipment
3. silo: a storage structure
4. silage: forage or animal food stored in a silo
5. toxic organic dust syndrome: a set of symptoms such as fever, headache, and malaise that occur after inhalation of dust in a silo or grain bin

Completion:

1. rural
2. June, July, August
3. traumatic
4. life threats
5. trained personnel
6. wash, hands
7. parallel
8. operator error

Completion:

S salivation, drooling
L lacrimation, tearing
U urination
D defecation, diarrhea
G GI distress, abdominal pain
E emesis, vomiting
M muscle contractions, twitching

1. SLUDGEM represents a set of symptoms common to exposure to organophosphate insecticides used on farms.
2. The treatment for exposure is atropine.

Short Answer:

1. entanglement, being struck, crush
2. heavy timbers for cribbing, heavy-duty air bags, or high lift jacks, front-end loaders, tow trucks, personnel from the local farm equipment dealership, physician, helicopter, all-terrain vehicles

Critical Thinking:

1. Dead birds at the chutes
2. brownish stains along walls
3. No, they may become victims themselves.
4. This rescue should be coordinated by a confined space rescue team familiar with silos.

Appendix A

Identification:

X An unconscious patient in respiratory distress with an OPA in place
__ A patient who states that it hurts to breathe
X A pulseless and apneic patient
X An unresponsive patient who has taken an overdose of narcotics
__ A seizing patient with a paramedic expected to arrive in 5 minutes
__ A patient who is choking on meat but is coughing forcefully
__ A patient with facial injuries who has gagged on an OPA
X Driver in a car versus tree collision; CPR in progress

Matching:

1. k
2. f
3. m
4. l
5. b
6. h
7. e
8. a
9. g
10. d
11. i
12. n
13. j
14. c

Definitions:

1. pneumothorax: air in the pleural space, potentially causing collapse of the lung
2. hyperventilate: to breathe faster and deeper than usual
3. aspiration: a term meaning to draw into; refers to foreign material inadvertently being drawn into the airway during an inspiration
4. tension pneumothorax: air in the pleural space under tension, causing complete collapse of the affected lung and shift of the heart, and other intrathoracic structures
5. direct laryngoscopy: using a laryngoscope to directly visualize the airway structures
6. endotracheal intubation: placement of a plastic tube into the trachea

True or False:

1. F
2. T
3. T
4. F
5. F
6. T
7. F
8. F
9. F
10. T

Ordering:

1 Assess patient
8 Lift blade upward and visualize the cords
12 Ventilate and confirm placement
9 Place distal end of tube through the opening between the cords
13 Secure tube and reassess patient
4 Assemble and test equipment
3 Place OPA and hyperventilate the patient
10 Remove blade
7 Place blade into right side of patient's mouth and sweep the tongue left
2 Lubricate and place stylet
6 Place patient in sniffing position (provided there is no trauma)
5 Stop ventilation
11 Instill air into the pilot balloon and remove syringe

Short Answer:

1. Visualization means the operator actually watches the tube pass between the vocal cords.
2. In auscultation, the operator hears air movement over both lungs, but not over the epigastrum (stomach).
3. When an aspirator is used, air is easily withdrawn from the trachea, but not from the esophagus. Stomach contents may be withdrawn from the esophagus.
4. A CO_2 detector indicates pressure of the carbon dioxide produced during metabolism. It will register high on air from the lungs, but very low on air from the stomach.
5. When the tube is correctly placed, patient assessment will show improvement in skin color.

Short Answer:

1. The letters stand for those things that should be considered if the patient is not responding well after intubation.
   D stands for displacement of tube.
   O stands for obstruction of the tube.
   P stands for pneumothorax.
   E stands for equipment failure.
2. You should deflate the balloon, remove the tube, and continue BLS ventilation of the patient.
3. You should ensure the balloon is deflated, remove the tube, and continue BLS ventilation of the patient.
4. Pull the stylet back so it is one-half inch above the Murphy eye.
5. Deflate the balloon, pull the tube back slightly, reinflate the balloon, and reassess for breath sounds over both lungs.

Critical Thinking 1:

1. The EMT-Bs must begin with BLS airway and breathing maneuvers. Position the patient. Open, assess, suction, and secure the airway. Begin ventilation with a high concentration of oxygen.
2. Ensure that there was good chest rise with ventilations and continue.

3. Provide the paramedics with the reason for the EMS call, initial assessment, changes in the patient condition, BLS treatment, and the patient response.
4. The EMT-Bs must have oxygen, a BVM, and suction. If carried, they should also bring in the intubation equipment.

Critical Thinking 2:

1. They should perform a jaw thrust and then begin suctioning.
2. They need to perform all BLS airway skills, but also consider an endotracheal intubation.
3. Have another EMT hold stabilization of the head and neck, while the first EMT performs the intubation. Do not place the head in the sniffing position.

Appendix B

Definitions:

1. **sudden cardiac death:** an unexpected death within 1 hour of the start of cardiac symptoms
2. **look, listen, feel:** a set of three steps to check for breathing; look for chest rise, listen for the sound of breathing, and feel for a breath against the cheek
3. **Heimlich maneuver:** forceful upward abdominal thrust designed to relieve a foreign body airway obstruction
4. **advanced lividity:** pooling of blood in dependent portions of the body
5. **return of spontaneous circulation:** pulses returning with just CPR or with defibrillation
6. **rigor mortis:** a generalized stiffening of the body
7. **signs of circulation:** responsiveness, breathing, coughing, and movement
8. **quick check:** opening the airway, checking for breathing, and feeling for a pulse simultaneously

Short Answer:

1. CPR is indicated if the AED advises no shock. It is used for arrest secondary to drug overdose, submersion in cold water, and hypothermia.
2. Any of the indicators of obvious death: rigor mortis, lividity, decapitation, incineration, decomposition
   Mortal wounds
   Do not resuscitate orders
3. First call or shout at the patient, then tap on the shoulder or finally deliver a painful stimulus.
4. Use the head tilt/chin lift if there is no suspected neck injury.
5. Adequate breathing
6. The carotid artery is found in a groove created by the sternocleidomastoid muscles along the side of the Adam's apple.
7. A child's head is larger than an adult's head, proportionally making it easy to close off the airway when the child is lying flat. In infants, the EMT should check a brachial pulse because it is difficult to palpate a pulse in the infant's neck. Compression and ventilation ratios follow the infant/child's vital signs; faster compression ratio and more breaths per minute.

Critical Thinking:

1. A selection of airway devices, suction, oxygen, bag-valve-mask, and an AED
2. Many answers are acceptable including the crowd, traffic, pets, and weather conditions.
3. Laypersons may look for signs of circulation rather than checking for a pulse, may omit ventilations and perform chest compressions only, and usually do not utilize other equipment except for a public access defibrillator/AED. EMTs would utilize supplementary oxygen, ventilation and airway devices, and move the patient toward an ambulance while continuing treatments.
4. They should assess scene safety, receive a quick report from the citizen as to what happened and what he has been able to do already. If the citizen is performing appropriate chest compressions and is willing to continue, they may utilize him thus freeing one of them to perform other procedures. They should utilize their AED and plan to move the patient toward the ambulance. Afterward, they may wish to thank the citizen for assistance while being careful not to violate confidentiality.

Appendix C

Definitions:

1. laryngoscope: tool used to visualize the glottic opening
2. hyperventilation: faster-than-normal rate of ventilation
3. cricoid pressure: partially occludes the esophagus, reducing the amount of air placed into the stomach during ventilation

4. twelve-lead ECG: a collection of 12 different views of the heart's electrical activity
5. normal saline (NS): the most common IV fluid; consisting of salt and water
6. D5W: 5% dextrose in water; consisting of sugar and water
7. macrodrip: allows for rapid administration of fluid
8. lactated Ringers solution (LR): used in same situations as NS; it is an electrolyte fluid
9. microdrip: used for delivering less fluid to a patient
10. preoxygenation: oxygen is delivered to the patient prior to intubation

Ordering:

1 Check the solution for clarity and date.
3 Remove the tab from the solution, and the cap from the drip chamber.
2 Select IV tubing size, open the packaging, and close the roller clamp.
6 Open the roller clamp and allow the fluid through the IV tubing.
4 Put the tubing spike into the appropriate IV solution port on the IV bag.
5 Hold the solution upright, and squeeze the chamber to fill the drip chamber halfway with fluid.

Short Answer:

1. Key "Do Nots"
   Do not recap a needle
   Do not stick a needle into a seat or mattress
   Do not throw a needle
   Do not throw away sharps in anything but an approved container
2. Ways in which an EMT can help an ALS provider to intubate:
   Apply cricoid pressure, allowing the vocal chords to come into view more easily, also reducing the amount of air being pushed into the stomach
   Preoxygenate the patient, prior to the arrival of ALS
   Provide suctioning of the airway, so that the ALS provider can see the chords
   Secure the endotracheal tube (ETT) after intubation
   Confirm ETT placement by listening to lungs and epigastric sounds
   Hyperventilate the patient for 30 seconds just prior to an intubation attempt
3. Right arm
   Left arm
   Right leg
   Left leg
   V_1: 4th right intercostal space at sternal border
   V_2: 4th left intercostal space at sternal border
   V_3: between V_2 and V_4
   V_4: 5th left intercostal space midclavicle line
   V_5: 5th left intercostal space anterior axillary line
   V_6: 5th left intercostal space midaxillary line
   See Figure C-7 in your text.